# Analytical Models Decision Making

D0514100

Colin Sanderson and Reinhold Gruen

Open University Press

Open University Press
McGraw-Hill Education
McGraw-Hill House
Shoppenhangers Road
Maidenhead
Berkshire
England
SL6 2QL

email: enquiries@openup.co.uk
world wide web: www.openup.co.uk

and Two Penn Plaza, New York, NY 10121-2289, USA

First published 2006

A catalogue record of this book is available from the British Library

ISBN-10: 0 335 21845 8 (pb)
ISBN-13: 978 0 335 218 455 (pb)

Library of Congress Cataloging-in-Publication Data
CIP data applied for

Typeset by RefineCatch Limited, Bungay, Suffolk
Printed in Great Britain by Bell & Bain Ltd., Glasgow

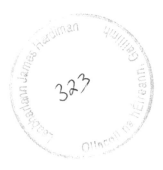

# Contents

# Acknowledgements

Open University Press and the London School of Hygiene & Tropical Medicine have made every effort to obtain permission from copyright holders to reproduce material in this book and to acknowledge these sources correctly. Any omissions brought to our attention will be remedied in future editions.

We would like to express our grateful thanks to the following copyright holders for granting permission to reproduce material in this book.

| | |
|---|---|
| p. 18 | Bensley DC, Watson PS and Morrison GW, 'Pathways of coronary care – a computer-simulation model of the potential for health gain', Mathematics Medicine and Biology, Vol 12, pp315–28, 1993, by permission of Oxford University Press. |
| pp. 155–6 | S Cropper and P Forte (eds), Enhancing Health Service Management, © 1997, Open University Press. Reproduced with the kind permission of Open University Press. |
| p. 68 | Cushman M and Rosenhead J, 2004, 'Planning in the face of politics: reshaping children's health services in Inner London' in Brandeau M et al (eds), Handbook of Operations Research and Health Care. Springer Science + Business Media. |
| p. 192 | Doll et al, British Medical Journal, 2004, Vol 328, pp 1519–1528. Reproduced with permission from the BMJ Publishing Group |
| pp. 133–6 | Reprinted with permission from Elsevier (The Lancet, 1999, Vol 353, pp1304–9) |
| pp. 52–4 | Gains A, and Rosenhead J, LSEOR Working Paper 93.8 'Problem structuring for medical quality assurance', LSEOR, 1993 |
| p. 167, 175 | Gruen RP, Constantinovici N, Normand C and Lamping DL, 'Costs for dialysis for elderly people in the UK', Nephrology Dialysis Transplantation, 18, 2122–2127, by permission from Oxford University Press. |
| pp. 1–6 | Lane D, Monefeldt C & Rosenhead J, Looking in the wrong place for healthcare improvements: a system dynamics study of an accident and emergency department, 2000, Journal of the Operational Research Society, reproduced with permission of Palgrave Macmillan |
| pp. 18–20 | Luckman J and Stringer J, 'The operational research approach to problem solving', British Medical Bulletin, 1974, 30, 257–261, by permission of Oxford University Press. |
| pp. 57–59, 93 | Rational analaysis for a problematic world revisited, Rosenhead J and Mingers J (editors). 2001, © John Wiley & Sons Limited. Reproduced with permission. |
| p. 137 | Sanderson C, 'Limitations of epidemiological needs assessment: the case of prostatectomy,' Medical Care, 35:669-85 by permission of Lippincott Williams and Wilkins. |
| pp. 24–6 | Sterman J, Business dynamics: systems thinking and modelling for a complex world, 2000, Mc-Graw-Hill Education, reproduced with permission of The McGraw-Hill Companies. |
| p. 171 | Soderlund Neil et al, British Medical Journal, 1997, Vol 315, pp1126-1129. Reproduced with permission from the BMJ Publishing Group |

p. 190, 210     Sonnenberg FA and Beck JR, Markov models in medical decision making: a practical guide, Medical Decision Making, 1993, Vol 13, issue 4, pp322–338

p. 104, 105–7   Thornton JG, Lilford RJ, Johnson N, British Medical Journal, 1992, Vol 304, pp1099–1103. Reproduced with permission from the BMJ Publishing Group

# Overview

## Introduction

Health care systems are complex. As a result, it is often unclear what the effects of changes in policy or service provision might be, whether on system performance or on the well-being of those needing care. There may be many objectives to be met and many interest groups to be considered. If public money is being spent, there should be public benefits, and these are hard to measure. All these factors mean that health care managers and planners have to make difficult decisions. At the same time, resources for health care tend to be in short supply, even though the benefits that they can provide are fundamental, so health care managers have a particular responsibility for making decisions well. This means making decisions that draw on sound information and judgement, and can be explained and justified.

## Why study analytical models for decision making?

There are methods of quantitative and qualitative analysis that can help decision makers to structure and clarify difficult problems, and to explore the implications of pursuing different options. These methods can draw on 'hard' and 'soft' information, and can be participative, explainable and justifiable. Models are diagrammatic and symbolic representations of problems. Some of these models are developed using more or less formal group processes. Many of them can be 'run' on personal computers to explore different scenarios.

The underlying concepts and ideas in this book are drawn primarily from the field of operational research (OR) which is the use of scientific methods to support management decision making and problem-solving. OR approaches have been developed and applied in a wide variety of contexts in the private and the public sectors. This is a very large and often technical field. The aim of this book is to provide you with a broad evaluative survey of the concepts and some hands-on experience with models, rather than expertise in specific techniques. By the end, you should be able to recognize the value of using analytical models to support decision making, understand and describe the strengths and weaknesses of some of the different types of model and approaches to analysing decisions, and choose analytical approaches appropriate to a particular situation.

This book will help you to think in an analytical way about some of the decision problems that you have to resolve; to carry out simple analyses of your own, but to recognize situations in which calling in experts may prove informative and how to make the best use of them; and to evaluate proposals and project reports by professional analysts, and articles in management or scientific journals. It will provide you with the basis for developing more specific interests and skills in the field, should you wish to do so.

## The structure of the book

There are 12 chapters grouped into four sections. Each chapter includes:

- an overview
- a list of learning objectives
- a list of key terms
- a range of activities
- feedback on the activities
- a summary

The book helps you build some simple models of your own and, on your CD-ROM, provides you with other models to try out. To build and run these models you will need to use a computer that has spreadsheet software which can read Microsoft Excel version 5 (or later) files for a PC, and can read a CD-ROM.

Some of the Excel features that you need to know how to use are:

- data entry using the formula bar
- moving around a worksheet using the mouse, scroll bars, and cursor keys
- selecting rows, columns, and cells
- formatting data
- inserting rows, columns, and cells
- moving data using cut, copy, and paste
- deleting data
- using formulae
- using functions
- using relative and absolute cell references
- displaying data as a chart
- formatting a chart
- sorting data in ascending or descending order
- using the drawing tools

You may well already be familiar with these. If not, learning about them will give you a skill that is well worth acquiring and which can be used in many different areas of public health. There are many comprehensive and well-illustrated books available on Excel, and there is extensive on-screen help built in to the software. You will not be expected to use or write macros, although of course you may do so if you wish.

You will find that some of the case studies and examples refer to the National Health Service in the UK. The methods are generic and can be applied to many different settings but you should think carefully about how they might need to be adapted before using them in your own work.

The following descriptions of the section and chapter contents will give you an idea of what you will be reading about.

### Section I Models and decision making in health care

In Chapter 1 you are introduced to the concept of a decision support model, to some different types of model, and to what makes a 'good' model. Chapter 2 takes you through a model-building process, from its conception to its validation and use.

Quantitative modelling and decision making methods commonly assume that there is a shared and reasonably good understanding of how systems work, and consensus about objectives among the various stakeholders. This is often not the case. This has led to the development of qualitative 'problem-structuring' methods, and in Chapter 3 you learn about one of them. Once a problem has been structured, it may be fairly obvious what to do, or it may then lend itself to a more quantitative approach.

## Section 2 Methods for clarifying complex decisions

The next three chapters are concerned with ways of clarifying decision problems. One way in which decisions can be difficult is that there may be many objectives or criteria, some or all of which may be ill-defined or conflicting. In Chapter 4 you learn about some methods of dealing with this. Another source of difficulty is uncertainty about how each option would perform in terms of your objectives, and in Chapter 5 you learn about different kinds of uncertainty and ways of handling them. In some circumstances it is possible to estimate the probabilities of different outcomes and in Chapter 6 you learn about how you can build these into a decision analysis.

## Section 3 Models for service planning and resource allocation

In Chapter 7 you learn about methods for estimating the level of provision required for a service of a particular type, using information on the characteristics of the population and on the effectiveness and acceptability of treatment. In Chapter 8 you learn about how to work out a feasible and acceptable balance of services where there are limits on the availability of resources. In Chapter 9 you learn about models for estimating the likely consequences, primarily in terms of costs, of changing patterns of hospital activity. (This chapter could also have been in the next section; it is about models used for planning and resource allocation, some of which involve evaluating possible changes in flows through systems.)

## Section 4 Modelling for evaluating changes in systems

System models describe how people, patients or other 'entities' flow between service providers and/or between states of health. These models are used to evaluate the effects on costs and outcomes of proposed policies, or changes to how the system operates. In Chapter 10 you start by learning about steady flows in static systems and go on to methods for modelling dynamic systems, i.e. systems which 'react' to attempts to change them, usually through self-stabilizing mechanisms. In Chapter 11 you consider fluctuating flows, which create problems in striking the balance between over-capacity leading to resources being under-used, and under-capacity leading to queues. Finally, Chapter 12 provides a brief review of what you have learned.

## Acknowledgements

The authors would like to thank Wayne Thompson, who played a major role in writing an earlier version of this book, and Jonathan Rosenhead, Emeritus Professor of Operational Research at the London School of Economics for use of the material on audit in Chapter 3, and for his many helpful suggestions. We are also grateful to Hannah Babad, Zaid Chalabi and Leon Garcia for testing the activities from a reader's point of view and to Deirdre Byrne for her support and help as manager of the series of which this is a part.

# SECTION I

# Models and decision making in health care

# The role of models

## Overview

In this book you will learn about a range of approaches to model building and decision support. The aim of this chapter is to introduce the main underlying concepts. You start by reading about types of rationality and what makes management decision making in health care difficult. You are then introduced to some of the different types of models that can be used to support and inform decision making processes, and read about a particular example of model building in health services. After this you learn about some of the components of a decision support model, and what makes a good model.

## Learning objectives

**By the end of this chapter, you will be better able to:**

- describe some of the characteristics of decision making in health care systems
- explain what is meant by a 'model' in the context of decision making, and identify the common features of such models
- describe some of the kinds of problem that health services models can help with
- understand the basic model-building process, what makes a good model, and some of the criticisms of using them to inform decision making

## Key terms

**Models** Ways of representing processes, relationships and systems in simplified, communicable form. Iconic models are representations of how the system looks. Graphic models are essentially diagrams, often consisting of boxes and arrows showing different types of relationships. Symbolic models involve sets of formulae, representing the relationships between variables in quantitative terms.

**Operational research (OR)** The application of scientific methods to management decision making. The development and use of symbolic, and more recently, qualitative models are arguably the distinctive features of the OR contribution.

**Problem structuring** Methods of clarifying problems by developing a shared understanding of them among decision makers or stakeholders, and clarifying objectives and options. They draw on ideas about procedural as well as substantive rationality.

**Procedural rationality** An approach to decision making that stresses reasoning processes and procedures for taking decisions when capacities to process information, and to forecast and compare outcomes are limited.

**Sensitivity analysis** Systematic exploration of how the outputs or results of a model change when the inputs, such as data and assumptions, are changed.

**Substantive rationality** An approach to decision making represented by: recognizing the need for a decision; clarifying the objectives for a 'good' outcome; identifying possible courses of action; assessing these courses of action; and choosing the 'best' course of action.

**'What-if ?' analysis** A process in which the decision maker, analyst and model interact, exploring the implications of different decisions under different scenarios.

## Introduction

Why is management decision making in health care difficult? To answer this question, you need to think about a more fundamental question: what makes a management decision a 'good' one? More broadly, how can you tell whether a decision made on behalf of an organization or group is a 'good' one? One obvious test is whether the decision can be justified: whether there are good reasons for it. This has led to the widespread acceptance of the idea that decisions should be made 'rationally'. But what does this actually mean? There are large and controversial economic, management, philosophical and psychological literatures on this that can only be touched on here.

One clear but demanding version of rationality requires:

1   an explicit set of options, or possible courses of action;
2   information that allows prediction of the outcomes of choosing each option; and
3   an explicit criterion for choosing the preferred set of outcomes, which is determined by the decision maker's goals and objectives.

The rational choice is the option that logic and the laws of probability suggest will lead to the best or most preferred set of outcomes. This, which Herbert Simon (1976) described as *substantive* rationality, is the basis for much economic theory (which assumes that 'economic man' actually is rational in this sense) and analysis (which assumes that decision makers should be). Indeed, substantive rationality lies behind many of the methods described in this book, particularly Decision Analysis in Chapter 6, where the aim is to maximize 'subjective expected utility'. However, Simon argued that in many practical situations decision makers cannot be sure of identifying the best option. Obtaining the necessary information may be impossible – or too costly, time-consuming, risky or unethical. Even if decision makers have the information, they may not have the capacity to process it; and even if they have the capacity, their preferences may change over time. Also while this approach, if feasible, leads to 'optimal' outcomes for individuals in a competitive context, it is not obvious what to do in a more collaborative world or if there are several decision makers with different preferences. Thus, the best that most decision makers can do is work with 'bounded' rationality, bounded that is by the complexity of the world they live in and their limited capacities for analysing it.

An objection to any version of rationality that is based solely on seeking good outcomes is that the means by which the outcomes are achieved may also be important. There are many versions of the story about the sheriff who could prevent a riot, in which thousands would certainly be killed, by framing and executing an innocent man (e.g. Smart 1973). In this case an exclusive focus on outcomes would require behaviour that is unethical, to say the least. There are ways round this, for example, by limiting the range of options to ethical ones, or expanding the outcomes to include the good standing of the law enforcement system, but the point remains.

One possible alternative to substantive rationality is *procedural* rationality. Here the test is not whether the best outcome is achieved, but how closely the decision making process follows particular rules or procedures. These procedures may be part of the institutional culture, such as rules of thumb that have produced 'good' decisions in the past. On the other hand, the justification for these procedures may be based on an appeal to accepted social principles such as transparency, rights and participation. Most writers on the subject have avoided being prescriptive about what makes a 'good' procedure, arguing that this depends on the context. But for priority-setting in health care, for example, Martin et al. (2003) describe a procedure that is justified in terms of: (1) how far it is driven by factors that fair-minded people agree are relevant; (2) its public accessibility; (3) whether there is a mechanism for appeal; and (4) whether adherence to the first three items is audited. This is based on a framework by Daniels (2000). In Chapter 3 you will read about a process designed to explore the implications for strategic action if the stakeholders have different points of view. The point is that in procedural rationality the option chosen is the one that emerges from a justifiable procedure. In contrast to substantive rationality, calculating or estimating the expected outcomes is not an essential step. 'Substantive rationality stresses rational choice, and procedural rationality stresses rational choosing' (Pidd 2004).

Simon's view was that substantive rationality was still the ideal, but suggested that where it is impossible, decision makers may *satisfice*. Instead of setting out to define and evaluate every option, decision makers may identify and evaluate successive options until they find one that meets a set of pre-specified standards. This option is then chosen because it is 'good enough', even though it has not been shown to be the best. Arguably this has elements of both substantive and procedural rationality, and Amartya Sen (1995) has shown that it is impossible to maintain a strict boundary between the two.

How do these concepts of rationality relate to the world of management? Mintzberg (1974) studied managerial work and drew a number of conclusions that have been summarized by Pidd (2004) as follows:

1 Many senior managers work long hours at an unrelenting pace.
2 Their activity is characterized by brevity, variety and fragmentation with constant switching between tasks.
3 The managers in the sample seemed to prefer the more active elements of their workload and disliked tasks such as reading mail and reports even though they might contain 'hard' data.

4  Linked to the point about activity, most of the managers seemed to prefer verbal media when communicating with people. The verbal communications were almost all about gaining and giving information, often soft information.

The picture is of continuous activity, of rapid decisions and consultations with individuals, together with longer scheduled meetings that involve many people. Throughout this activity, the manager is continually receiving and sifting information, seeking out that which is relevant now or which might be useful in the future. It is not an image of a life of detached, contemplative reason.

It is this milieu of continuous activity, of rapid decisions and consultations with individuals, that defines the bounded rationality employed when making strategy and developing policy.

This illustrates some of the constraints and pressures found in managers' working environments. What about the nature of the problems that they have to address? In 1979 Ackoff argued that:

> Managers are not confronted with problems that are independent of each other, but with dynamic situations that consist of complex systems of changing problems that interact with each other. I call such situations messes. Problems are abstractions extracted from messes by analysis; they are to messes as atoms are to tables and chairs. Managers do not solve problems; they manage messes.

More recently, Pidd (2004) set out some of the more specific challenges to good *strategic* decision making along the following lines:

1  Instead of a smooth annual planning cycle, threats and opportunities may arise which require a rapid response under pressure.
2  There may be confusion and disagreement about objectives. Working out *how* to do something can be hard enough, but in strategic decision making the questions are more often *what* should be done and *why*.
3  The leaders of any organization have generally emerged as the leaders because they are good at getting what they want. Strategic debate can involve struggles between powerful people.
4  Most organizations have plenty of operational data, which enable it to operate more or less efficiently in its present form and context. However, the challenge in much strategic decision making is to find ways to deal with the new and unknown.
5  Strategic decisions are often complex as well as very important. They may involve many different factors and interactions between factors, so that making a change to one will have consequences elsewhere. These decisions involve human beings who may construe the same situation quite differently from one another.
6  Planners are rarely in full control of the situation. Other actors, such as competitors, legislators and customers will also affect what happens. The organization must find ways to roll with that future so as to achieve some goal.

To complete this introductory section on rationality in decision making, here are some brief extracts from an article by the sociologist Amitai Etizioni (1986) in which he proposes an alternative to the notion of the ever-rational 'economic man'.

This article examines the merits of the notion that . . . rationality is anti-entropic. That is, the 'normal' state of human behaviour is assumed to be non-rational; for behaviour to be rational even in part, forces must be activated to pull it in the rational direction. Moreover, following such an activization, behaviour 'strives' to return to the entropic state . . .

The 'normal' state is one in which behaviour is not purposive, non-calculative, governed by emotions and values, potentially inconsistent and conflict-ridden, indifferent to evidence, and under the influence of 'group-think' (i.e. individuals defer in their thinking to group-defined facts, interpretations, and conclusions even if they diverge significantly from objective reality.) . . .

It will become evident that because rationality is artificial, i.e. manufactured, it has a cost.

 **Activity 1.1**

In the light of what you have just read and your own experience, under what circumstances can substantive rationality be a practical basis for decision making?

 **Feedback**

Substantive rationality becomes more practical:

- the clearer and less controversial the set of priorities and objectives
- the better defined the set of options or actions
- the better understood or more predictable the relationships between actions and outcomes
- the less extensive the trade-offs between competing objectives

 **Activity 1.2**

In your view, to what extent do these conditions prevail in health care? In brief, what evidence do you have to support your view?

 **Feedback**

Health care organizations consist of many different interest groups (for example, different types of health care professionals, policy makers, managers) and are made up of many small organizational units. Each group and unit may have its own aspirations and objectives, and with so many different interest groups it is often difficult to establish a clear set of overall priorities and objectives.

It can also be difficult to define a set of decision options when the decision 'environment' is turbulent. In health care, managers have to contend with continual change in medical technology, in methods of service delivery, in management arrangements, in health policy, in human resource policies, in funding available, in patterns of disease, in patient expectations, etc.

Evaluating decision options in terms of their capacity to achieve organizational objectives is also difficult in health care. The relationships between health care activity and
health improvement, for example, are often obscure. With growing investment in
research and information systems, this situation has been improving, but there will
always be an element of uncertainty.

In short, health care is a difficult environment for substantive rationality. It is not
straightforward for procedural rationality. On the other hand, it is widely accepted that
health is important, both as an end in itself and as a means to other ends; that health
care is important to health; and that there is room for improvement in health care
decision making. This makes the question of how to improve health care decisions
difficult but important.

## The contribution of OR and management science

The problem of how to make management decisions in the context of uncertainty,
controversy and turbulence is clearly not unique to health care. Contributions
have come from people with a wide variety of professional and academic
backgrounds – management and social scientists, mathematicians, operational
researchers, economists – working in industry, commerce, defence and
government.

The main stream of the earlier theoretical work in operational research and
management science (OR/MS) was very much within the 'substantive rationality'
paradigm. It was devoted to methods of analysis and optimization: ways of describing the system in question, predicting the likely impact of choosing specific
options and choosing 'best' solutions. However, among practitioners there was less
emphasis on sophisticated mathematical methods and more on developing a good
understanding of the problem with decision makers and 'what-if ?' analyses, in
which analysts and decision makers interact, exploring the implications of different
decisions in a wide variety of scenarios.

More recently the domains of both theory and practice have drawn closer together,
and the importance of procedural rationality has been more explicitly recognized.
The result has been the development of a number of approaches to the following:

- *problem structuring* – ways of clarifying problems by developing a shared
  understanding of them among decision makers or stakeholders, and clarifying
  objectives and options;
- *decision support* – ways of identifying the information needed on options and
  effects on outcomes, and organizing and processing it in a way that leads to
  appropriate decisions, thus extending decision makers' capacities to process
  information.

The central concept in both of these is the *model*, and the rest of this chapter will be
devoted to exploring some of the ideas underpinning model development and
evaluation.

## Types of model for decision support

A typical definition of a model might be along the lines of:

> a model is a simplified representation or description of a system or situation, used to improve understanding or decision making.

This definition is rather different from common usage of the word. A dictionary might also suggest something like:

- an ideal or a standard to be imitated (for example, a model student)
- a physical representation on a different scale (for example, a model aeroplane).

It might be argued that the second two definitions are special cases of the first. Managers may wish to develop a 'model' service on paper as a simplified expression of their vision, for the purposes of communication and leadership. Reduction in scale will mean some loss of detail or function and thus simplification, but a model aircraft may be useful for the purposes of, say, wind-tunnel testing and improving design. However, for the purposes of problem structuring and analysis, you will mainly be concerned with understanding and describing how a system actually works – correctly identifying the factors that determine whether your objectives are achieved, and how these factors operate – as a basis for decisions about what to do.

Of course, models of this kind are not only used in decision support. Scientists of many kinds use models to explain and predict phenomena even though they may have no intention of trying to change them. Table 1.1 summarizes some of the main differences between decision-driven and knowledge-or evidence-driven modelling.

**Table 1.1** Evidence-driven and decision-driven model building

|  | Evidence-driven | Decision-driven |
|---|---|---|
| Starting point | What can we find out about X? | What should be done about X? |
| Task | Learn from synthesis of data | Explore policy options and futures |
| Inputs | Scientific evidence | Science + expert opinion if need be |
| Outputs | Understanding of causal chains | Pros and cons of options |
|  | Inconsistencies/implications of data | Robustness of outcome to scenarios |
|  | Important gaps in knowledge | Important gaps in knowledge |

Next you will examine, in very broad terms, some of the common features of such models and some of the main types of models used in health services management.

Models for decision making are primarily of three types:

- iconic
- graphic
- symbolic or mathematical.

### Iconic models

Iconic models show the physical or spatial relationships between objects. They generally look like what they are meant to represent but are different in scale. The model aeroplane is an example. Most such models are used for communication of ideas but maps are examples of iconic models used in decision making. For example, a plan of a railway system shows the physical interconnections between stations. Its purpose is to help passengers decide which lines to use and where to change trains so as to get from one station to another. However, it is a model in the sense that it is a highly simplified representation of the system, designed for a specific purpose. Typically it does not show other information that might be useful, such as costs and travel times, the length of the connecting walkways between platforms, distances to a car park or town centre, etc.

## Graphic models

Graphic or conceptual models are essentially diagrams showing relationships (usually represented as arrows) of a non-spatial kind between a set of elements (usually represented as boxes). It is useful to distinguish between representations of the following:

- logical sequences of activities
- influences or effects (inter-relationships between variables)
- flows of objects between elements of a system
- systems (flows + effects)

### Logical sequences of activities

Logic (or planning) models show the links between the various activities that may be involved in the achievement of an objective. The aim of such a model is usually to develop and communicate a plan or schedule. Figure 1.1 is a very basic example. The overall task is broken down into a number of more specific activities which are represented by boxes or 'nodes'. Arrows between nodes indicate the order in which the activities should be carried out. There are no strict conventions however. In a variant widely used for project management and known as the Critical Path Method, arrows represent activities and nodes represent events. Logic diagrams of this kind are also used in the design of computer systems and programmes.

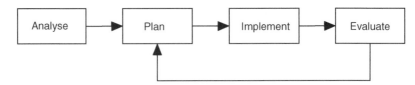

**Figure 1.1** A logic model for planning

Here the sequence of links is essentially *prescriptive* ('how to do it'), although there might also be evidence to suggest that this approach is effective. In practice, models of this kind range from the very broadly conceptual, such as Figure 1.1, to the extraordinarily detailed network charts used in the construction industry.

### Influences or effects

Here the task is to capture and convey an understanding of how a system works and why. Influence diagrams show chains of cause and effect, with a view to informing decisions about how to change or influence an 'outcome' variable. The boxes represent variables and the arrows show which variables affect, or are affected by, which. Figure 1.2 shows a very simple example of an influence model used for health promotion.

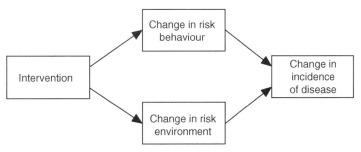

**Figure 1.2** An influence model for health promotion

Some of the cause–effect relationships involved may be based on empirical evidence, while others may be matters of theory or belief. However, the intention is generally to be descriptive, so it is important to be clear about which links in the chain are speculative or controversial, and it may be necessary to investigate these further before deciding on what action to take.

### Flows

In flow models the boxes typically represent processes and the arrows show how entities being processed (such as patients being treated) flow from one process to another. Figure 1.3 provides a simple example. The interest here is usually in understanding how the different elements in a system contribute to the performance of the whole and in managing the system's capacity. Again, the intention is generally to be descriptive.

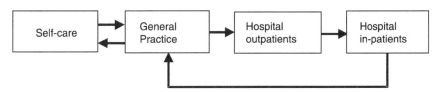

**Figure 1.3** A patient flow model

### Systems

System models are essentially combinations of flow and influence models. To avoid confusion between arrows which represent flows and arrows which represent influences, some sort of convention is needed. In *system dynamics* diagrams, for example, flows are represented by double-sided straight lines evocative of water pipes, and influences by single curving lines. Figure 1.4 shows Lane and colleagues' (2000) system dynamics model of an accident and emergency department and how it links into the larger system, including scheduled admissions and the hospital wards. You will learn more about models of this kind in Chapter 10.

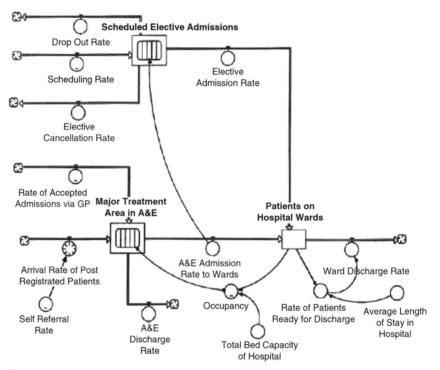

**Figure 1.4** A system model

Source: Lane et al. (2000).

## Symbolic or mathematical models

The main value of graphical models is in developing and communicating a qualitative understanding of a system or situation. Sometimes this will allow an assessment of the decision options that is good enough to determine an appropriate course of action. Many decision-support models start life in graphical form. But if quantitative answers are needed to 'what-if' questions, it is necessary to go further and build a symbolic or mathematical model.

Instead of boxes and arrows, these consist of sets of mathematical expressions, with symbols representing variables. For example, Clarke and Clarke (1997) and others have used 'gravity' models in health systems planning for estimating the effects of changes in hospital capacity on flows of patients to it and to other hospitals nearby. One form of gravity model is as follows:

$$T_{ij} = M_i * C_j * B_j * e{-}\text{ß}_j \, d_{ij}$$

for

$T_{ij}$ = estimated patient flow from zone $i$ to hospital $j$

$M_i$ = relative morbidity of population in zone $i$

$C_j$ = capacity of hospital $j$

$B_i$ = scale factor to match total flows from zone $i$ to hospitals with the 'need' in zone $i$

$d_{ij}$ = distance of hospital $j$ from population in zone $i$

$\text{ß}_j$ = deterrence parameter representing how flows to hospital $j$ decline with distance

This expression quantifies the extent to which people tend to use nearby and distant hospitals.

To convert a graphic model into a mathematical one you will typically need one such expression for each arrow leaving a box. For an influence diagram these expressions indicate the strength of the effects that 'input' variables (arrows into the box) have on 'output' variables (arrows out). For a flow diagram these might indicate how the volumes of flows out of each service point depends on the flows into it, and a systems model will involve expressions that represent how these volumes of flow depend on combinations of flows in and influences.

Figure 1.5 shows a 'pathways-of-care' diagram used in modelling the impact of a heart disease prevention programme. Here a graphical (boxes and arrows) model has been supplemented by numerical information on the nature and scale of the flows. As long as the percentages involved remain constant, this information provides the basis for a simple type of mathematical model; it can tell you something about what is likely to happen to the flows to specialist medical treatment for example, if the annual number of new cases of angina increases. This model has been used as a means of communicating to non-clinicians the flow of patients between different health states and treatments, and also by health authorities to evaluate different purchasing options in a series of 'what-if' calculations.

## A health services management model

The following extract from Luckman and Stringer (1974) describes how a management model helped to solve a problem in health care. At this stage all you need to take from this extract is a broad idea of what they were trying to do.

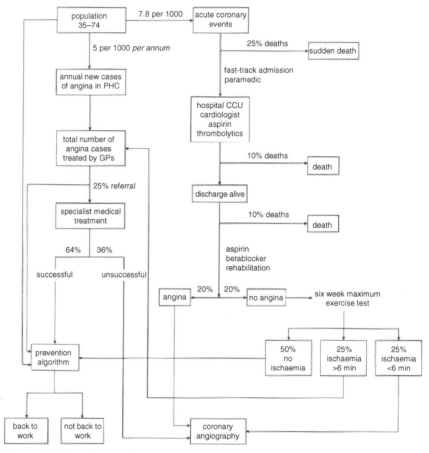

**Figure 1.5** The pathways of coronary care
Source: Bensley et al. (1995).

### A simple example of the operational research process

The nature of OR is first explained by reference to one of the most straightforward cases, namely that of a single decision making group intent upon achieving results of a certain kind but faced with alternative courses of action which they might employ to achieve their purpose. It is also implicit that the alternatives are too numerous, or that the relation between action and effect is too complicated, for the choice to be obvious. The steps that might be taken towards making a rational decision could be set out as follows:

1  recognition of the need to make a choice;
2  identification of courses of action available;
3  definition of the desired objective;
4  consideration of the extent to which the desired objective would be achieved by each available course of action;
5  choice of the course of action which seems best;
6  implementation of the chosen action.

Although OR might be concerned with helping at any of these stages, it is at steps (4) and (5) that the most characteristic feature of OR, the creation and use of a model, occurs.

The following example, which has been discussed more fully elsewhere, is repeated here in outline to demonstrate the use of a model. The decision making group consisted of a senior administrator, a matron and a senior member of the medical staff of a large general hospital for acute diseases. Their problem in essence concerned the provision of an Intensive Therapy Unit within the hospital, although since the group were already committed to the idea, the decision problem was more in terms of how large a unit should be provided. The courses of action open to the group were numerous, since the choice of size of the unit mentioned in previous debate had ranged from two beds to 24 beds. The OR approach in this case was to estimate the likely demand for care in such a unit, and to this end a survey of patients throughout the hospital was mounted. The decision making group were involved from the outset, first, in clarifying the criteria by which patients requiring intensive therapy could be identified and, second, by formulating, with the help of the research team, the most useful ways of expressing objectives. This latter problem was reduced to a discussion of the compromise that would be necessary between having too few beds – with resultant lack of the specialized treatment on a number of occasions – or having too many beds – with a high level of care but with some expensive resources being inefficiently used. In the end, it was agreed that potential solutions to the problem should be judged on the basis of the level of service, i.e., the proportion of the required days of care that could be offered by the unit. The decision making group chose a level such that no more than one in 500 patients needing care should find the unit full.

The model, based on data collected in the survey, was simply a mathematical representation of the flow of patients into and out of a hypothetical unit over a reasonable period of time. The model results matched the actual incidence of the care required by patients in the survey, and it was then possible to proceed to postulate different courses of action and to measure the extent to which the desired objective would be achieved. For example, with the level of care required by the patients in the survey, seven beds were found to be necessary to meet the objective that no more than one in 500 patients should find the unit full.

At this stage, however, one further element must enter the discussion. The process of introducing change in a system made complex by the involvement of human behaviour as well as by purely technical matters may well alter some of the factors affecting the behaviour of the system. Although we have little precise knowledge of how behaviour may change, it is often necessary to consider, as we did with the decision making group, some of the likely responses to change that may result. Such matters as the nursing response to the presence of the unit (perhaps a tendency to keep patients in the unit for longer than strictly necessary), the likely changes in demand (the attraction of the unit over a larger catchment area once the unit has been established), and changes in such factors as length of stay and death rate were all discussed, and estimates were put forward by the group members.

A fresh look at the model was made with the revised estimates and it was demonstrated that the provision of eight beds would meet the desired objective. Furthermore, the sensitivity of this solution to grosser changes in the factors was explored by use of the model. For example, if the demand or the average length of stay doubled, 10 beds would be required to provide the same level of service. Hence the result is relatively insensitive to quite large changes in these factors. Note also that because of the non-proportional change in need with demand, the more usual method for assessing the number of beds, based on a fixed proportion of the total number of hospital beds, would be in error.

The group chose the eight-bed solution as being best for their purpose and this was the action that was later implemented.

 **Activity 1.3**

Now answer the following questions. (You will probably need to go back and read parts of the text more carefully.)

1   The decision making group used a model to forecast the number of beds required in an Intensive Therapy Unit (ITU). Are there any other aspects of the decision making process for which the model was or may have been useful?

2   Why did the decision maker favour using a series of 'what-if' calculations to obtain a robust estimate of the behaviour of the system rather than finding the optimum solution?

3   There are a number of features that decision-support models, iconic or symbolic, have in common:

  (a) *Outcome variables* – the variables that represent how far the decision makers have achieved their objectives.

  (b) *Exogenous variables* – variables that can affect outcomes directly or indirectly, but which are not affected by other variables within the model. In symbolic models their values are based directly on data, assumptions or pre-defined scenarios.

  (c) *Intermediate or endogenous variables* – variables in the model that link the exogenous variables to the outcome variables. In symbolic models their values are calculated from values of exogenous and/or other endogenous variables.

  (d) *Control variables* – variables that can affect outcomes and are under the decision makers' control or influence.

  (e) *Structure* – the elements in the model that can be assumed not to vary over the time horizon of interest, such as the variables in the model, which variables are related and, in symbolic models, the formulae relating them.

Can you identify these in the ITU model?

 **Feedback**

1  The ITU bed model was also useful in the following ways:

  (a) in establishing a shared understanding of the problem between members of the decision making group

  (b) in communicating ideas about the decision making problem: clarifying the objectives and possible options for action

  (c) in identifying the necessary input data

  (d) in exploring the number of beds required, assuming different 'what-if' scenarios.

2  The complexities of systems in health care mean that model builders are often unsure about how well their model represents the real world. They may not have

identified or included all the important factors. There may be insufficient data about the factors that they *have* identified and about how one part of the system affects another. These problems make it difficult to be sure that the best decision according to the model will be the best in the real world. Instead of picking the decision that works best with the model, it will often be safer to identify a *robust* decision that is satisfactory over a range of scenarios.

3 (a) *Outcome variables* – these are implied in the objectives of avoiding 'too few beds – with the resultant lack of specialized treatment on a number of occasions – or having too many beds – with a high level of care but with some expensive resources being inefficiently used'. The decision makers want to maximize 'the proportion of the required days of care that could be offered by the unit' but, by implication, they also want to take into consideration the occupancy of the unit. These objectives are in conflict and the task is to find a good balance between them.

(b) *Exogenous variables* – One is 'the need for care in such a unit'. Another possible exogenous variable is length of stay in the unit. This is certainly part of the model, although you have to be sharp to spot this; it only appears in passing in the last paragraph ('if average length of stay doubled'). In this case it seems to have been treated as an exogenous variable (nurses may have 'a tendency to keep patients in the unit for longer than strictly necessary') but if the nurses had been involved in the analysis, it might have become a control variable.

(c) *Intermediate or endogenous variables* – This is a simple model which involves no intermediate variables. In a larger model, with 'survival of severely ill patients' as its outcome variable, 'percentage admitted to intensive care' could have been an intermediate variable.

(d) *Control variable* – 'choice of size of the unit'

(e) *Structure* – Here the essential elements of structure are a stream of patients arriving with needs for care; a unit with a fixed number of beds; and stays in the unit of determinable length and variability.

## Types of model

You have just been reading about a model of an Intensive Therapy Unit. When you looked at the contents page of this book you may have noticed that the different chapters were not characterized by the field of activity involved (maternity services, population screening, etc.) but by more abstract features of the situation. This is because there are 'families' of models that can be applied in a variety of different circumstances.

A critical factor in successful use of models in decision making is choosing the appropriate form of model. For example, you will learn about applications of the following types of model later in this book:

- *Game-theory models* for decision making under 'uncertainty', that is when the future values of the relevant exogenous variables or 'states of nature' cannot be estimated, even in probabilistic terms (Chapter 5).
- *Decision analysis models* for when probabilities can be attached to each potential future value of the relevant exogenous variables or 'state of nature' (Chapter 6).

- *Programming models* for estimating the effects on efficiency of changes in the way mixes of resources are allocated to tasks (Chapter 8).
- *Costing models* for predicting the effect on costs and performance of changing factors such as case mix and service capacity (Chapter 9).
- *System dynamics models* for predicting how the effects of decisions will unfold over time, particularly when there may be vicious or virtuous circles of cause and effect, leading to stable or unstable behaviour of the system as a whole – or parts of it (Chapter 10).
- *Queuing models* for where the rates of arrival at an interconnected system of services, or the service times themselves, are irregular. These models provide estimates of the effect on measures of performance (waiting times, occupancy) of changes in service capacity or scheduling arrangements (Chapter 11). The intensive therapy unit you have just read about would have been one of these.

## Building 'good' models

If they [models] were as complex and difficult to control as reality there would be no advantage in their use. Fortunately we can usually construct models that are much simpler than reality and still be able to use them to predict and explain phenomena with a very high degree of accuracy. The reason is that although a very large number of variables may be required to predict a phenomenon with perfect accuracy, a small number of variables will usually account for most of it. The trick, of course, is to find the right variables and the correct relationships between them.

(Ackoff and Sasieni 1968)

How can you tell whether a model can predict and explain phenomena with sufficient accuracy for your purpose? Of course, this will depend on the purpose. In a problem-structuring exercise, the emphasis may be on explanation and clarification rather than prediction. However, models are often used to explore the outcomes of pursuing different options and in these cases some sort of predictive validity is important.

A model is in a sense the embodiment of a set of theories, and ideally models should be tested or validated according to similar principles. It follows that estimates or predictions made using the model should be tested against observed reality. Poor fits indicate problems with the model, which need to be investigated and remedied. As the number of 'good enough' predictions begins to grow, so does confidence in the model, although strictly any model can only be provisional. Counter-intuitive predictions that turn out to be correct can be particularly persuasive. A number of cycles of data collection, calculation, validation, and modification may be required. Once there is sufficient confidence in the model it can be used to explore the possible outcomes of different combinations of management decisions and scenarios. This in turn can be used to inform decision making, although usually there will be factors that are outside the model to be taken into account. Figure 1.6 is a representation of this process.

Unfortunately for many decision support models, predictive validation of this kind may not be possible because, for one reason or another, it is not possible to collect suitable test data before the decision has to be made. For the kinds of

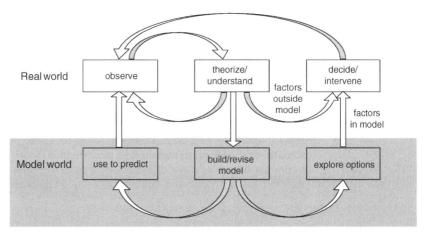

**Figure 1.6** A graphic model of the model-building process

decision that have to be made repeatedly, it might be worth investing in developing and testing a model over a number of decision cycles. But even then, there is still the problem of the 'counterfactual': how do you *know* what would have happened if a different decision had been taken? Hodges and Dewar (1992) take a strong line on this:

> Few military models or models of human decision making can be validated, and it is counterproductive to demand as a matter of policy that users and institutional parents attempt to validate them . . . [A] model that cannot be validated in the [predictive] sense is not necessarily useless; it simply may not be used to make sentences like 'the model says X'.

This is a problem that cannot be ignored. Weinstein et al. (2001) suggest five evaluation criteria which can be applied when tests of predictive validity are impracticable:

- *Transparency*: are the assumptions, input parameters and the logic connecting them to outputs, stated with complete clarity and are they open to peer review?
- *Verification*: are the outputs of the model consistent with observed data? Has the model been debugged and tested for internal consistency?
- *Corroboration*: have other models of the same problem produced similar results contingent upon similar assumptions and input parameters?
- *Face validity*: do the results of the model make sense in relation to theoretical considerations?
- *Accreditation*: has the model been subjected to peer review by a dispassionate reviewer and found to be what it claims to be?

There are other considerations worth mentioning here.

- *Parsimony*: Einstein is credited with saying 'A model should be as simple as possible, *and no simpler.*' Again, there is an implication of fitness for purpose; for example, decisions involving a long-term perspective may require more complex models than short-term decisions.
- *Robustness*: conclusions should not depend on unreliable data or assumptions.

Sensitivity analysis should have been carried out to assess the robustness of the model's predictions to changes in suspect parameters.

- *Accessibility/flexibility*: the model should have a 'friendly' interface, which makes it easy for the user to understand the nature of the model, to make changes in parameters and to obtain different kinds of analyses.
- *Relevance*: the model should be able to address the important questions. This may seem an obvious point but there are many different types of model and many modellers who specialize in a particular type; there may be specialist software involved, for example. Naturally, if asked by a decision maker to model a particular situation, specialists will tend to use their own type of model. This may not be the most relevant approach.

More insights into what makes a good model and a good decision making process can be gained from some of the criticisms of model building. There are two main threads. The first relates to practicality and cost.

- *Models can be over-ambitious*. This, again, is perhaps more a criticism of modellers than models. It is tempting to try to construct a general model that can be used to address a wide variety of circumstances and questions. However, this can lead to loss of focus on any particular issue, unrealistic requirements for data, and extension of the development phase to the point that the model is either not ready in time or out of date as soon as it is ready.
- *Models require too much data*. This criticism is a variant of the first. However, models can have a useful role in identifying which items of data are worth seeking out or collecting.
- *Models cost too much to develop*. Model building can be seen as part of the cost of the decision making process, and the cost of making a decision needs to be related to what is at stake. The effort involved needs to be proportionate to the amount gained by making good as against bad decisions. This may be affected by how far the decisions in question are irreversible or costly to reverse.

The second type of criticism is that models place too much power in the hands of experts and technocrats, marginalizing legitimate stakeholders and adding obscurity rather than transparency to decision making. It is true that, like many potentially powerful tools, models can be abused. On the other hand, they are, by definition, explicit, and so *in principle* available for scrutiny, criticism and improvement. Their explicit nature also offers a basis for accountability which, while not always comfortable for decision makers, is a desirable characteristic when decisions are being made by a group of managers on behalf of others – such as a community of tax payers or insurance payers. To counter this kind of criticism, models need to be fully documented and open to scrutiny. However, the situation may be complicated by commercial considerations and issues regarding the protection of intellectual property.

This chapter will end on a provocative and prescriptive note, with an extract from a book by John Sterman (2000).

 **Business dynamics: systems thinking and modelling for a complex world**

The word validation should be struck from the vocabulary of modelers. All models are wrong, so no models are valid or verifiable in the sense of establishing their truth. The question facing clients and modelers is never whether a model is true but whether it is useful. The choice is never whether to use a model. The only choice is which model to use. Selecting the most appropriate model is always a value judgment to be made by reference to the purpose. Without a clear understanding of the purpose for which the model is to be used, it is impossible to determine whether you should use it as a basis for action.

Models rarely fail because the modelers used the wrong regression technique or because the model didn't fit the historical data well enough. Models fail because more basic questions about the suitability of the model to the purpose aren't asked, because the model violates basic physical laws such as conservation of matter, because a narrow boundary cut critical feedbacks, because the modelers kept the assumptions hidden from the clients, or because the modelers failed to include important stakeholders in the modeling process.

To avoid such problems, whether as a modeler or model consumer, you must insist on the highest standards of documentation. Your models must be fully replicable and available for critical review. Use the documentation to assess the adequacy of the model boundary and the appropriateness of its underlying assumptions about the physical structure of the system and the decision-making behavior of the people acting within it. Consider extreme condition tests and sensitivity to alternative assumptions, including assumptions about model boundary and structure, not only sensitivity to variations in parameter values.

Model testing is iterative and multidimensional and begins at the start of the project. Build into the budget and time line sufficient resources to assess the impact of the work and to document it fully so others can help you improve it.

No one test is adequate. A wide range of tests helps you understand the robustness and limitations of your models. These tests involve direct inspection of equations and simulations of the whole model, the assessment of historical fit, and behavior under extreme conditions.

Use all types of data, both numerical and qualitative. Multiple data sources provide opportunities for triangulation and cross-checking.

Test the robustness of your conclusions to uncertainty in your assumptions. While parametric sensitivity testing is important, model results are usually far more sensitive to assumptions about the model boundary, level of aggregation, and representation of decision making. Test as you go. Testing is an integral part of the iterative process of modeling. By continuously testing your assumptions and the sensitivity of results as you develop the model, you uncover important errors early, avoid costly rework, and generate insights throughout the project, thus involving your clients more deeply and building their – and your – understanding of the problem and the nature of high leverage policies.

Open the modeling process to the widest range of people you can. Implementation success requires changing the clients' mental models. To do so the clients must become partners with you in the modeling process. Ultimately, your chances of success are greatest when you work with your clients to find the limitations of your models, mental and formal, then work together to correct them. In this fashion you and your clients gradually develop a deep understanding of the system and the confidence to use that understanding to take action.

Design assessment into your work from the start so you can determine both the extent to which you meet your goals and how you can improve the process in the future. Work with your clients to collect data that can reveal how your work affected the beliefs, attitudes, and behavior of the people in the system, along with changes in system performance. Track the impact of your work with long-term follow-up studies. A careful testing and assessment process helps you and your clients improve your ability to think systemically in every aspect of your lives, not just in one project.

## Summary

You have seen that decision making in health care is complex. There will be uncertainty about the environment and about activity by other organizations, controversy about objectives and uncertainty about the relationships between control, exogenous and outcome variables.

You have seen that there are many different types of models in health services management and that models can be used not only to inform decision making but also in clarifying and arriving at a shared understanding of a problem. You should recognize some of the common features of models and have some preliminary ideas about what makes a good model.

This chapter has been a rather abstract introduction to some of the thinking behind decision-support models. In the next chapter you will go through the process of building a model of your own.

## References

Ackoff RL (1979) The future of operational research is past. *Journal of the Operational Research Society* 30: 93–104.

Ackoff RL and Sasieni MW (1968) *Fundamentals of Operations Research*. New York: Wiley International.

Bensley DC, Watson PS and Morrison GW (1995) Pathways of coronary care – a computer-simulation model of the potential for health gain. *IMA Journal of Mathematics Applied in Medicine and Biology* 12: 315–28.

Clarke G and Clarke M (1997) Spatial decision support systems for health care planning, in S Cropper and P Forte (eds) *Enhancing Health Services Management*. Buckingham: Open University Press.

Daniels N (2000) Accountability for reasonableness. *British Medical Journal* 321: 1300–1.

Etzioni A (1986) Rationality is anti-entropic. *Journal of Economic Psychology* 7: 17–36.

Hodges JS and Dewar JA (1992) *Is It You or Your Model Talking? A Framework for Model Validation*. RAND, R-4114-AF/A/OSD.

Lane D, Monefeldt C and Rosenhead J (2000) Looking in the wrong place for healthcare improvements: a system dynamics study of an accident and emergency department. *Journal of the Operational Research Society* 51: 518–31.

Luckman J and Stringer J (1974) The operational research approach to problem solving. *British Medical Bulletin* 30: 257–61.

Martin D, Shulman K, Santiago-Sorrell P and Singer P (2003) Priority-setting and hospital strategic planning: a qualitative case-study. *Journal of Health Services Research and Policy* 8: 197–201.

Mintzberg H (1974) *The Nature of Managerial Work*. New York: HarperCollins.

Pidd M (2004) Contemporary OR/MS in strategy development and policy making: some reflections. *Journal of the Operational Research Society* 55: 791–800.

Sen A (1995) Rationality and social choice. *American Economic Review* 85: 1–24.

Simon HA (1976) From substantive to procedural rationality, in HA Simon (ed.) *Models of bounded rationality: behavioural economics and business organization.* Cambridge, MA: MIT Press.

Smart J (1973) An outline of a system of utilitarian ethics. In J Smart and B. Williams *Utilitarianism: For and Against.* Cambridge: Cambridge University Press.

Sterman JD (2000) *Business Dynamics: Systems Thinking and Modeling for a Complex World.* Boston: Irwin McGraw-Hill.

Weinstein MC, Toy EL, Sandberg EA et al. (2001) Modeling for health care and other policy decisions: uses, roles and validity. *Value in Health* 4: 348–61.

## Overview

In this chapter you will work through the design and analysis of a model of a highly simplified health care programme which covers three diseases. You will start by developing a graphic model of the causal links that allow the programme to achieve its objectives. You will then use this to develop a symbolic model and then estimate the number of lives saved for different balances of expenditure between the three diseases, to help decision makers choose the best balance. This chapter brings together all the stages of the model-building cycle that you learned about in Chapter 1.

## Learning objectives

**By the end of this chapter, you will be better able to:**

- **formulate and build a qualitative model to address a decision making problem in managing a community health care programme**
- **simplify and refine the model structure**
- **identify and gather relevant data**
- **build a spreadsheet model**
- **use the model to predict the impact of different options in terms of the number of lives saved**
- **carry out sensitivity analyses**
- **evaluate the model**

## Key term

**Marginal return** The additional benefit secured for an additional amount of expenditure. In general, marginal return diminishes with increasing expenditure.

## Introduction

Models are abstractions and Chapter 1, which was about models in general, was very abstract indeed. Now you are going to build a model of your own. This chapter is loosely based on a health care management game originally developed by Creese and Gentle (1974).

A team of local health care managers has a budget to cover the costs of treatment in their population. Their overriding concern is with preventing as many premature deaths as possible. Prevention of the onset of disease is beyond their scope: in other words, they cannot influence the incidence of the disease in the population. What they can do is treat people with existing disease. This is a highly simplified scenario to introduce you to the process of developing and using a model for decision support.

Your tasks will be to:

- represent the programme with a graphic model or influence diagram
- simplify the graphic model to provide the basis for a symbolic model
- seek relevant data
- build a symbolic model using a spreadsheet and the data available to you
- estimate the costs and numbers of lives saved for different patterns of activity
- carry out a sensitivity analysis for dubious data or assumptions
- evaluate your model.

Note that 'lives saved/£' will be used as a shorthand for 'premature deaths prevented per unit of expenditure on treatment'.

## Step 1: Draw up an initial graphic model

First, think about what the managers are trying to achieve. They want to save the maximum number of lives with their given budget (or equivalently, minimize the costs per life saved). This suggests it would be helpful to have a model that could predict the lives saved/£ for different patterns of health care activity. So lives saved/£ is your *outcome* variable.

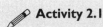 **Activity 2.1**

Your first task is to identify the factors that may influence your outcome variable. Draw an influence diagram showing the relevant factors for *one disease*. You may find it helps to start with your outcome variable on the right of a sheet of paper and work 'upstream' to the left, first, identifying the direct or 'proximal' influences (intermediate variables such as numbers treated and effectiveness of treatment) and then moving on to the indirect or more 'distal' factors such as the severity of case mix in the population that in turn affect your proximal influences. (The higher the proportion of those with the disease in the population that have severe symptoms, the more severe the case mix and the greater the risk of death.) At this stage, include any factors you think might be influential. Simplification comes later. At the same time, do stick to the agenda. Your immediate concern is with saving the maximum number of lives with a given health care budget, not with preventing morbidity, promoting equity or community benefit.

Once you have formulated your model, identify the *control* variables, the factors that the managers can decide upon or influence relatively directly, and indicate them on your diagram.

The managers are concerned with saving lives, so you can define a 'treatment impact factor' as the difference in case fatality between treated and untreated cases. Of course, not all patients with a particular disease have equal potential to benefit.

In mild cases the untreated case fatality may be very low. Suppose it is 5 per cent. If treatment reduces the case fatality to zero, the treatment impact factor in this group would be 5 − 0 = 5 per cent.

For more severe cases, the untreated case fatality rate might be around 50 per cent. If the case fatality among treated cases were 30 per cent, the treatment impact factor would be 50 − 30 per cent = 20 per cent. You can assume that the more severe the disease, the greater the treatment impact factor. This is only an approximation to reality, as the practice of 'triage' implies.

Some of the relationships that you might include in your model at this stage are:

*   'Numbers of lives saved' depends on the numbers treated and their treatment impact factors.
*   Treatment impact factors depend on the severity of the case mix and quality of care.
*   Quality of care depends on factors such as staff training and clinical audit systems.
*   Costs of treated cases depend on fixed and variable costs.
*   Fixed and variable costs depend on numbers of patients treated and the efficiency of the care providers. Efficiency is related to quality of care.
*   Severity of case mix is related to the numbers of patients treated. First priority is given to the most severe cases, so as the proportion of all prevalent cases that are treated increases, more mild cases are treated, and the case mix becomes less severe.
*   The numbers of cases of each disease treated depends on guidelines and indications for treatment.

## Feedback

Figure 2.1 shows one version of such a model. It may look complicated but there is nothing very profound about it and it still lacks detail. You may have gone into more detail in some areas and less in others, or included different factors altogether, or shown different types of relationships between them. There are many valid ways of representing the same situation. Comparing and discussing differences between different people's graphic models can be very instructive.

To understand Figure 2.1, try starting on the right and working backwards, or 'upstream' through it. For example, it implies that the cost of treated cases depends on the fixed and variable costs of treatment, and the numbers of lives saved depend on the numbers of patients treated and their treatment impact factors. (Note: in Figure 2.1, 'complementary services' are other services which are not formally part of health care but which, like community services for the elderly or disabled, fill complementary supportive roles, and so may affect the scope of what has to be done *within* the health care system).

In principle, the factors that the health care managers can influence might include health care policies (which influence indications for treatment and thus numbers treated), and quality of care (which influences costs and effectiveness). In Figure 2.1 these are shown as double-edged boxes.

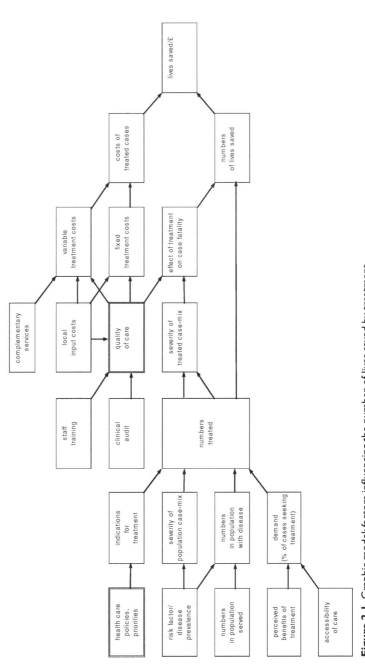

**Figure 2.1** Graphic model: factors influencing the number of lives saved by treatment

## Step 2: Refine the graphic model

The next step is to refine your model in the light of what has been learned about the system and the managers' concerns so far. After some discussion, the managers decide that they will not be able to change the treatment impact factors and costs of treatment in the short term, and that the best prospect for making improvements in output is by changing the mix of activity – i.e. treat more people who would benefit more, and fewer people who would benefit less. In this population there are only three diseases (A, B and C) and the question becomes how many people with each disease to treat. Decisions about which individual patients to treat are made by a large variety of people and involve many considerations, so this will be a matter of strategic direction rather than micro-management.

You may be able to leave factors out if they are expected to be unchanged over the time scale for which the model is meant to be valid. Remember that if exogenous variables are expected to vary, some attempt will have to be made to forecast *how* they might vary.

You may also need to add more detail, however. Now that the focus is more clearly on strategic management of the balance of numbers treated for each disease, you should make sure that all the relevant effects of changing this balance are included.

 **Activity 2.2**

Your task now is to refine your graphic model for one disease and use it as a basis for devising a *symbolic* model that can predict the number of lives saved for different numbers treated. You should introduce appropriate notation or symbols for your variables. Then you should derive formulae showing how the outcome variable can be calculated from the control and exogenous variables. Don't spend too much time on this and move on to the Feedback if you get stuck. The important point here is to go through the various steps involved in constructing the model.

 **Feedback**

Figure 2.2 shows a revised version of the model shown in Figure 2.1. Remember that this is for just one disease. The control variable is $n$ (the number of cases of the disease in question that are treated) and the wholly exogenous variables are $p$ (prevalence) and $m_u$ (case-fatality in untreated patients). A number of factors have dropped out. You are not expecting changes in the quality of care, for example; case fatality for treated patients $m_t$ will be determined solely by case mix, and all the factors influencing quality of care can drop out. Also you do not expect changes in disease or risk factor prevalence, or in demand for care.

However, two new relationships have been added, indicated by dotted lines. On reflection it was realized that changing the numbers of patients treated would probably have effects on:

• *variable costs*: increasing treatment volumes might lead to lower costs per patient, partly through economies of scale and partly because it would lead to treating less severe patients as suggested above;

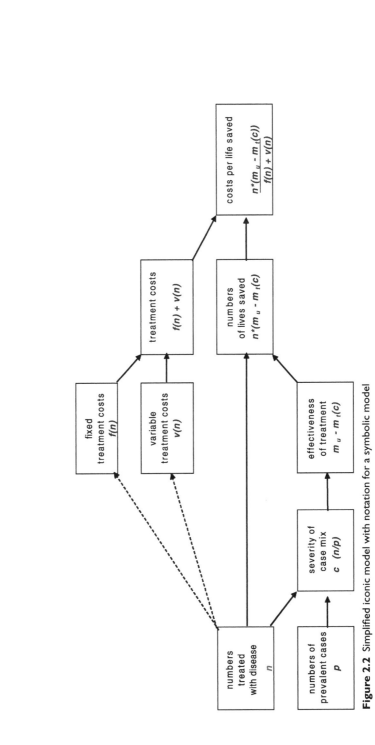

**Figure 2.2** Simplified iconic model with notation for a symbolic model

The boxes in the figure contain:

costs per life saved
$$\frac{n*(m_u - m_t(c))}{f(n) + v(n)}$$

treatment costs
$f(n) + v(n)$

numbers of lives saved
$n*(m_u - m_t(c))$

fixed treatment costs
$f(n)$

variable treatment costs
$v(n)$

effectiveness of treatment
$m_u - m_t(c)$

numbers treated with disease
$n$

severity of case mix
$c \ (n/p)$

numbers of prevalent cases
$p$

- *fixed costs*: depending on current levels of unused capacity, it could be that to increase patient volumes, investments would have to be made in new equipment or refurbishment.

Figure 2.2 shows the formulae for *intermediate* variables such as treatment costs, in keeping with the use of a graphic model to provide a means of communicating underlying ideas and methods.

Some points to note:

- Variable costs are shown as $v(n)$ because they depend on $n$ (the number treated), but at this stage you are not sure what this relationship looks like.
- Severity of case mix depends on the proportion of prevalent cases treated, $n/p$ where $p$ is the number of prevalent cases in the population, since priority is given to the most severe cases, and it is assumed that the *distribution* of severity is not affected by changes in prevalence.
- Lives saved are calculated using the difference between treated and untreated case fatality rates, $m_u(c) - m_t(c)$.

With the notation in Figure 2.2, the symbolic model becomes:

number of lives/£ saved by treating $n$ patients $= n*[(m_u(c) - m_t(c))]/[f(n) + v(n)]$

## Step 3: Identify and gather relevant data

A research organization is commissioned to assemble some relevant information and produces Table 2.1. This gives data on treated and untreated mortality, and on variable and fixed costs, for different levels of activity for each disease. Have a close look at these data. Remember that the expected treatment benefit per patient is the difference between the fatality rates for the treated and untreated groups:

**Table 2.1** Data for diseases A, B, and C

| Disease | Patients per year | Additional £000s to set up | per case | Mortality untreated (%) | treated (%) |
|---|---|---|---|---|---|
| A | 1–100 | 20 | 2.2 | 11 | 4 |
|   | 101–200 | 0 | 2.1 | 9 | 2 |
|   | 201–300 | 0 | 2.0 | 7 | 2 |
|   | 301–400 | 0 | 2.0 | 6 | 2 |
|   | 401–500 | 0 | 2.0 | 2 | 1 |
| B | 1–100 | 0 | 1.0 | 5 | 0 |
|   | 101–200 | 0 | 1.0 | 4 | 0 |
|   | 201–300 | 5 | 1.0 | 3 | 0 |
|   | 301–400 | 0 | 0.8 | 1.5 | 0 |
|   | 401–500 | 0 | 0.8 | 1.0 | 0 |
| C | 1–100 | 10 | 0.40 | 3.0 | 1 |
|   | 101–200 | 0 | 0.40 | 2.5 | 1 |
|   | 201–300 | 0 | 0.35 | 2.0 | 1 |
|   | 301–400 | 9 | 0.30 | 1.7 | 1 |
|   | 401–500 | 0 | 0.30 | 1.5 | 1 |

- Case fatality and treatment benefit per patient are expected to decline as the numbers of patients treated increase. That is because first priority is given to the most severe cases, who for these diseases are also those with the greatest potential to benefit.
- For disease A, the cost per case is expected to decline with increasing volume. There are no set-up costs for disease B at lower treatment rates but an extra lump of expenditure is needed if volumes rise above 200 per year, for some additional item of equipment. The same applies to disease C at levels above 300.

Notice that there are no data relating to severity of case mix; Table 2.1 shows how case fatality depends directly on numbers treated. Severity will have to be dropped as an explicit intermediate variable and the model simplified slightly so that

effectiveness = $m_u(n) - m_t(n)$ rather than $m_u(c) - m_t(c)$.

This means you will have to drop prevalence from the model as an exogenous variable. In what circumstances could this create problems? Suppose that the distribution of severity of disease A in the population shifts and the mean decreases. Then the severity of treated cases might decrease as well and the model will overestimate the numbers of lives saved by treating a given number of cases. However, unless there is some dramatic new method of primary prevention any such changes will be fairly slow and this should not be a serious omission.

How reliable are the data in Table 2.1? The cost estimates are based on local information and thought to be generally trustworthy. But there is some doubt about the case fatality data, as these are based on studies in the literature rather than local data. The figures for the least severe cases are particularly suspect, as they are based on small numbers of deaths. You make a note that you will need to do some sensitivity analysis, trying different values for these parameters to see how much they alter the conclusions.

On this basis you may be content with your model as it stands. But if not, you should take another turn around the model development cycle, re-examining your theory and/or collecting new data, in an effort to improve your model.

## Step 4: Build a spreadsheet model

You will now build a model using Excel. If you are not yet a confident Excel user, don't worry. Follow the instructions as best you can and if you get stuck look carefully at the model provided and described in the feedback that follows.

This is a strategic programme and the managers decide that it will be sufficient to determine the care programme strategy once a year, in multiples of 100 patients.

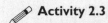 **Activity 2.3**

Type the data from Table 2.1 into a spreadsheet using columns C (e.g. C6:C20) and D for set-up and variable costs respectively. List them by disease and numbers treated, as in this table, and use columns E and F for untreated and treated mortality.

Calculate, for each disease:

- the marginal (i.e. additional) number of lives saved for each additional 100 patients treated (in column J)

- the marginal cost of each additional 100 patients (in column K)
- the lives saved/£100,000 for each block of patients treated (in column M).

Make sure you tidy up by putting in informative column headings and row labels before you move on.

If you know how to create an Excel chart, make one that shows the marginal rates of lives saved/£ for each disease, for each block of 100 patients.

### ↻ Feedback

The Excel workbook 'Ch2TreatProg' contains a completed worksheet for this activity called 'Calculations'. The figures in the yellow areas are the input data and figures in light blue area are derived from these, using formulae.

The formula in cell J6 given by = I6*(E6-F6)* comes from $n*(m_u - m_t)$ in your symbolic model. Formulae corresponding to J7 = (I7–I6)*(E7–F7) were put in the range of cells J7:J20 by using Copy and Paste. (You can trace the figures that feed into formulae by using the Excel Audit facility. Try this out by clicking on 'Tools' in the main menu across the top of the screen, then click on 'Formula Auditing' and then on 'Trace precedents'. To hide the arrows that this produces, click on 'Tools/Formula Auditing/Remove all arrows'.)

The formula for marginal cost in cell K6 is = C6+D6*I6, in K7 it is = C7+D* (I7–I6) and this was copied to the range of cells K7:K20.

The formula for marginal lives saved per £100,000 in cell L6 is = (J6*100)/K6, copied to the range of cells L7:L20.

If you made a chart, it should look something like Figure 2.3, with data on lives saved per £100,000 from column L.

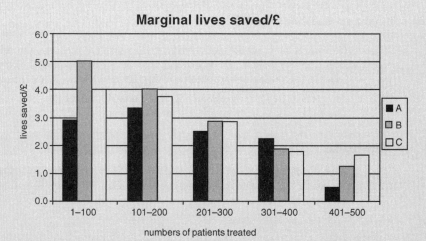

Figure 2.3 Lives saved/£ in each treatment programme

## Step 5: Use the model to decide on the strategic balance

The next step is to decide how many of each type of patient to treat. You have a total budget for these diseases of £1,000,000.

**Activity 2.4**

First, look at Figure 2.3. What general messages does this give you?

**Feedback**

From Figure 2.3, you should note the following points:

- For all these diseases, returns in lives saved/£ generally diminish with increasing activity. Thus, although there may be cost savings with increasing activity, these are outweighed by the less severe nature of the patients treated, who have lower capacity to benefit.
- For disease A the cost savings with increasing activity are more nearly balanced with declining benefits than for other diseases, so the returns are relatively constant across the range of up to about 400 patients treated per year. This level of activity seems sufficient to provide treatment for most of the patients who might derive significant benefit.
- The treatment programme for disease B is effective for the most severe cases but with increasing numbers (and declining severity) the marginal returns diminish more quickly than for A.
- At lower volumes the programme for disease C is costly because of the annual fixed costs but it is more cost-effective than disease A.

These findings may help decision making in qualitative terms but there is a little more work to do if you want to calculate the best allocation.

**Activity 2.5**

Now use your spreadsheet to calculate the best allocation.

**Feedback**

If your budget were only £100,000, you would save most lives by treating 100 patients with disease B, the tallest column in Figure 2.3. If you had another £100,000 in your budget you would add the second-highest column, etc. So it would be useful to rank the values in column L in order. Excel can do this for you. But remember that column L contains formulae and trying to sort formulae does not work. One way is as follows:

- Highlight cells H4:L20 so that you include row and column labels. Click on 'Copy'.

Highlight cell N4. Right-click on your mouse and choose 'Paste Special'. On the menu click on the 'Values' box and then 'OK'.

- You now have a copy of H4:L20, but with values instead of formulae. (Compare the contents of cells L6 and R6.)
- Now highlight N6:S20, and use Data/Sort. This brings up a menu page. Make sure that 'no header row' is clicked and then sort on column R 'descending'.

You now have the returns to each block of activity in descending order of benefit/£.

Finally, type 'spend' in S4 and put the formula '=S5+Q6' in S6. Then copy S6 into the range S7:S20. The results should look like the table in the rust-coloured area of 'Calculations' in the file 'Ch2TreatProg'.

This gives you the cumulative expenditure involved, so that if you carry out all the activity down to row 16, your expenditure will be given by cell S16. You can now see that if you had a budget of £1,000,000 and were treating in blocks of 100, you would save most lives by treating 200 cases of disease A, 300 of B and 300 of C. The estimated cost of this would be only £880,000, so you could also treat a number of patients from the next block of expenditure, which would be on A.

A word of warning: this 'ranked increments' approach only works if there are consistently diminishing (or more strictly, non-increasing) returns to increasing activity. If the untreated case fatality rate for the first 100 cases of disease A were 4 per cent rather than 3 per cent, the lives saved/£100k would be 2.9, less than the return for cases 101 to 200 of A (which is 3.3). The sorting method would suggest that you choose the block of cases of A from 101 to 200 *before* the block from 1 to 100, but this is impossible. In this situation you have to merge blocks until you do get diminishing returns. Taking cases 1 to 200 of disease A together gives an overall figure of 3.1, which can then take its place in the rankings. An alternative approach would be to use some kind of procedure or algorithm for searching through the possible combinations of expenditure, but this is beyond the scope of this chapter.

## Step 6: Carry out sensitivity analyses

Some people in the hospital may not be happy with these answers. How robust are they? Inspection of column R shows that the rankings, especially in the middle of the order, could easily be changed as a result of quite small changes in the estimated costs per case and case fatality rates. You need to investigate the effects on your results of errors in your data and changes in your underlying assumptions.

Remember that the researchers are fairly confident of the cost figures, since these are based on local data. They are less sure about the mortality data as these are based on published studies carried out in other hospitals. In this model the effectiveness of treatment is $(m_u - m_t)$, the difference between treated and untreated case fatality. The researchers have provided range estimates for this difference, since this is the only exogenous factor in lives saved. These are given in Table 2.2, which shows middle, upper and lower estimates for $(m_u - m_t)$.

**Table 2.2** Different estimates for the impact of treatment on case fatality

| Disease | Patients per year | Additional £000s to set up | per case | Case-fatality difference (%) mid | upper | lower |
|---------|-------------------|---------------------------|----------|----------------------------------|-------|-------|
| A | 1–100 | 20 | 2.5 | 8.0 | 9.0 | 7.0 |
|   | 101–200 | 0 | 2.4 | 7.0 | 8.0 | 6.0 |
|   | 201–300 | 0 | 2.0 | 5.0 | 6.0 | 4.0 |
|   | 301–400 | 0 | 2.0 | 4.0 | 4.5 | 3.0 |
|   | 401–500 | 0 | 2.0 | 1.0 | 3.0 | 0.0 |
| B | 1–100 | 0 | 1.0 | 5.0 | 6.0 | 4.0 |
|   | 101–200 | 0 | 1.0 | 4.0 | 5.0 | 3.0 |
|   | 201–300 | 5 | 1.0 | 3.0 | 4.0 | 2.0 |
|   | 301–400 | 0 | 0.8 | 1.5 | 2.5 | 1.0 |
|   | 401–500 | 0 | 0.8 | 1.0 | 2.0 | 0.0 |
| C | 1–100 | 15 | 0.3 | 1.5 | 2.5 | 1.1 |
|   | 101–200 | 0 | 0.3 | 1.0 | 1.7 | 0.7 |
|   | 201–300 | 0 | 0.3 | 1.0 | 1.7 | 0.5 |
|   | 301–400 | 9 | 0.3 | 1.0 | 1.7 | 0.5 |
|   | 401–500 | 0 | 0.25 | 0.5 | 1.0 | 0.3 |

### Activity 2.6

Suppose that the upper estimates in Table 2.2 were used for disease A, so that treatment for disease A was more effective than it was first thought to be, and the lower estimates for diseases B and C, so that treatment for these two diseases was less effective? How would this affect the best mix of activity? (Again, if you are unfamiliar with Excel, think how you might work this out and then have a look at the worksheet called 'Sensitivity 1'.)

### Feedback

This is a fairly extreme form of sensitivity analysis. The worksheet called 'Sensitivity 1' gives the results. This looks similar to the 'Calculations' sheet except that another column has been added to the table in the yellow 'Data' area and Table 2.2 has been copied into it.

Also, instead of one version of the tables in the blue 'Calculations' area and the red 'Results' area, there are three, based on different combinations of figures from Table 2.2, and labelled in column I. The results are as follows:

The best allocations are:

With upper estimates for A, lower for B and C:     300+ A, 200 B, 200 C

With upper estimates for B, lower for A and C:     200+ A, 400 B, 200 C

With upper estimates for C, lower for A and B:     200 A, 400 B, 400+ C

On this basis there seems no doubt that they should be doing at least 200 A, 200 B and 200 C. Beyond this, two of the scenarios favour 400 B.

### Multiple criteria and value judgement

This model assumes there is only one simple objective: maximizing the number of lives saved for a given budget. With just one objective, it is possible to calculate a 'best solution'. No judgements are involved. In reality, though, there will be other objectives. Treatment may be designed to prevent pain or disability as well as death. Also there may be equity issues; it may not be acceptable to focus on B and C and treat very few cases of A, even if this saved the most lives.

One question you might ask is whether changing the mix of activity really does make a large difference to the number of lives saved. If it does, using lives saved to decide on the best mix of activity might be a reasonable approach. But if changing the mix actually makes very little difference to the lives saved but makes a large difference to prevention of disability or even to numbers treated, you may be able to achieve a lot more benefits of other kinds if you were willing to accept a slight reduction in lives saved.

This question is examined in the worksheet called 'Sensitivity 2'. The calculations up till now have been made on the basis that allocations are 'lumpy'; they can only be made in blocks of 100 patients. Here, this crude approach is refined by:

- allocating as many blocks as possible within the budget;
- then allocating whatever fraction of the next block can be fitted within the budget, assuming that each patient within a block has the same variable treatment cost and risk of mortality.

If you are interested in how this was done, look at the table in the rust area of Sensitivity 2 called 'Budget allocation'. The number of 100s of cases of diseases A, B and C to be treated are placed in cells E24:E26. The disease that you want to use any unspent budget on is placed in B30. The resulting numbers of patients treated and lives saved are in E32 and F32, and these are copied by value into the table headed 'Summary of results'. Different combinations of numbers for A, B and C provide the different rows in the table.

This table exploits two useful Excel functions: MATCH(value, range) which scans the range for the best match to the value (as used in cell C30); and OFFSET(reference, rows, columns) which returns the value in a particular row and column in a table (as used in e.g. cells F24:F26). Thus OFFSET(A1,3,5) would return the contents of cell F4, because offsetting three rows from row 1 gives row 4, and offsetting five columns from column A gives column F. Use the Excel Help if you want to find out about what these do.

Table 2.3 gives some results for different ways of using the budget of £1,000,000. (The number of possible combinations is very large; these are just some of the best ones.) It turns out that with this budget the numbers of lives saved is fairly insensitive to the mix of activity. The top six options differ by about one life saved in 33. On the other hand, there are large variations in the numbers of patients treated, so that compared to the best option in terms of lives saved, another option would save one or two fewer lives but provide 226 more patients treated. It seems that the results of the model are at odds with the managers' perception that they could improve the lives saved/£ by changing the mix of activity.

In this situation, the best option will necessarily be *a matter of opinion*, depending

**Table 2.3** Sensitivity of lives saved and numbers of patients treated to activity mix

| Allocation (100s treated) | | | Lives | Number |
|---|---|---|---|---|
| A | B | C | saved | treated |
| 2.6 | 3 | 3 | 33.5 | 860 |
| 2.41 | 3 | 4 | 33.2 | 941 |
| 3.13 | 2 | 3 | 33.1 | 813 |
| 2.26 | 3 | 5 | 33.0 | 1026 |
| 2.93 | 2 | 4 | 32.9 | 893 |
| 2.78 | 2 | 5 | 32.6 | 978 |
| 1.86 | 4 | 5 | 32.2 | 1086 |
| 3.23 | 3 | 0 | 32.0 | 623 |
| 1.48 | 5 | 5 | 30.6 | 1148 |
| 4 | 1 | 1 | 30.5 | 600 |

on the relative weights given to avoiding death as against any other benefits from treating patients. Any decision may be based on a consensus but there may well be people who disagree.

The key point is that once more than one criterion is involved, there is no objectively best option unless one option is equal to or better than all others on all criteria.

## Step 7: Evaluate the model

 **Activity 2.7**

With the evaluation criteria set out in Chapter 1 in mind, what can you say about the scope for evaluating this model? (Remember that in this case the aim of building it was to take you through the steps in model building, rather than develop a model that would stand up to scrutiny as a basis for real decision making.)

 **Feedback**

In terms of *transparency*, simple spreadsheet models have the advantage that many managers are familiar with Excel, so they can examine the formulae and try the models out for themselves. This will give them a chance to assess *face validity* at least. Complex spreadsheets, or models based on general purpose programming languages such as Delphi or C++, need to be very well documented, and even then are difficult to understand for anyone but the model builder. The use of software written for special purposes, such as decision analysis or system dynamics, can help avoid programming errors and provide a friendly interface but may impose limitations on the kinds of question that can be addressed.

In terms of *predictive* validation, the results of this model can be tested for plausibility – whether they are in the right kind of range – but not for correctness. The main problem is with the case fatality rates. Suppose you decided to carry out a follow-up study to check the estimates of fatality in treated patients. Suppose further that you had prognostic indices good enough to sort the patients into blocks of 100 in terms of expected treatment impact factor. Even then, with case fatality rates of less than 10 per cent, there will be too few deaths in any one year to allow accurate estimates. The model values might fall within the confidence intervals derived from the observed data but this would not be a very discriminating test.

In terms of *accreditation*, models published in the scientific literature should have been subjected to dispassionate peer review. Publication also allows corroboration between different models in the literature. Some specialists and consultants have models that have been used in a variety of settings. Publication and repeated use with different decision makers in different situations may help build confidence in the model structure but both leave open the question of calibration to local circumstances.

To summarize, in the first of a series of cycles of decision making it may not be possible to use a model that has been validated against empirical data in the local context. It may be necessary to rely on consensus, internal logic and data from elsewhere.

## Summary

In this chapter you have developed a kind of theory about the factors that determine the number of lives saved (your initial graphic model), reviewed and selected from the relevant data that are available locally, and devised an initial simplified model based on these data. You went on to drop some variables because, on reflection, they were unimportant in the context of this problem. Including them in the initial model was not wasted effort on your part but a necessary part of the process of understanding the system. You also dropped some variables because there were no data available. It is good practice to think through the possible implications of this. It may be necessary to take steps (and the time and resources) to obtain new data, or include the variables in question and use estimates.

You then used your model to predict numbers of lives saved with different patterns of activity and to explore the sensitivity of your results to changes in your model.

You could have compared your model predictions with reality but in this case it would not have been conclusive because the numbers of deaths were small and volatile. You discussed your results with local experts and stakeholders, and the conclusion was that your model was sufficiently plausible to be useful.

You found that the initial assumption that changing the mix of activity might be a good way of increasing the numbers of lives saved was not supported by the model. Many combinations of activity mix saved about the same number of lives. However, the total numbers treated could be changed substantially by changing the activity mix. The question then was whether it was right to opt for many more patients treated if this meant giving up saving even a small number of extra lives. This is a question for the decision makers, not the model builder.

## Reference

Creese AL and Gentle PH (1974) Planning in district management: use of a teaching game. *Lancet* 2: 337–40.

# 3 | Strategic Options Development and Analysis

## Overview

In Chapter 1 you were introduced to procedural rationality and, briefly, to problem structuring methods (PSMs). There are several of these methods and in this chapter you will learn about one of them, Strategic Options Development and Analysis (SODA). This is a process through which people can achieve a consensus about, and commitment to, strategic action. You will consider the theoretical basis of this approach as well as its key technique, cognitive mapping, and study an application in the management of health services.

## Learning objectives

**By the end of this chapter, you will be better able to:**

- **outline the Strategic Options Development and Analysis approach and describe its use as a group decision support system**
- **draw a cognitive map**

## Key terms

**Cognitive mapping** A term from psychological research on perception which describes the general task of mapping a person's thinking. A cognitive map is not simply a 'word and arrow' diagram or an influence diagram; it is the product of a formal modelling technique with rules for its development.

**Strategic Options Development and Analysis (SODA)** A problem-structuring approach designed for working with messy problems. The aim is to facilitate the process by which a team arrives at consensus and commitment to action. The cognitive maps of each member of a client team are merged to form an aggregated map called a 'strategic map'.

**Strategic workshops** Part of SODA, these involve two 'passes'. The aim of the first pass is to begin the process of participants 'taking on board' alternative views and in the second pass, focusing on specific issues, the 'rules' change, discussion is encouraged and commitment to action is sought.

## Introduction

In Chapter 1 you learned how the main stream of the earlier theoretical work on models for decision support was very much within the 'substantive rationality' paradigm, devoted to predicting the likely impact of choosing specific options and choosing best solutions. However, among practitioners there was less emphasis on sophisticated mathematical methods and more on developing a good understanding of the problem and exploring a wide variety of scenarios. The past 20 years or so have seen the emergence of problem-structuring methods. More in tune with the idea of procedural rationality, these help group decision making by providing structure to the processes involved so that 'those who must take responsibility for the consequences of choices do so on a coherent basis' (Rosenhead and Mingers 2001).

The book which is the source of this quotation has had an important role in disseminating problem-structuring methods and the ideas behind them. The main methods include Strategic Options and Development Analysis (SODA), Soft Systems Methods (SSM), the Strategic Choice approach, Robustness Analysis, and Drama Theory. You will touch on Robustness Analysis and on one aspect of the Strategic Choice approach in Chapter 5. In this chapter you will learn about SODA.

## SODA

The following edited extract by Eden and Ackermann (2001) gives an introduction to the SODA approach and explains its core techniques of cognitive mapping, merging maps and strategic workshops.

 **Strategic Options Development and Analysis (SODA) – the principles**

With SODA the traditional model building and analysis skills of the operational researcher are used to . . . facilitate the better management of the process by which the team will arrive at something approaching consensus and both emotional and cognitive commitment to action. Underlying this notion of success is a view of problem solving that focuses on the point at which people feel confident to take action that they believe to be appropriate. This is in contrast to the idea of striving for the 'right answer'.

The SODA approach has its foundation in 'subjectivism'. Each member of a client group is held to have his or her own personal subjective view of the 'real' problem. The wisdom and experience of members of the team are a key element in developing decisions with which participants feel confident. It is because of the complexity and richness that arises from attention to subjectivity, that a focus for SODA work is on the managing of process as well as content. This view of behaviour, judgement and decision making in organizations sees experience-gathering as an act of 'scientific' endeavour, where managers experiment with their organizational world, learn about it, develop theories about how it works, and seek to intervene in it.

This *focus on the individual*, or on the *psychology and social psychology* of problem solving, is guided by the 'Theory of Personal Constructs' (Kelly 1955). This particular body of psychological theory is a cognitive theory. It argues that human beings are continually striving to 'make sense' of their world in order to 'manage and control' that world, and suits the particular purpose of working with individuals who are constrained by a need to explain their actions within their organizational world.

*Cognitive mapping for SODA*

'Cognitive mapping' is the label for the general task of mapping a person's thinking within the field of psychological research on perception. It is important to note that cognitive mapping is not simply a 'word and arrow' diagram, or an influence diagram . . . or a 'mind-map'/'brain-map' (Buzan and Buzan 1993). It is a formal modelling technique with rules for its development; without such rules it would not be amenable to the type of analysis expected of a formal model.

The term cognitive map was first used by Tolman in 1948, and has been used widely since then by researchers in a wide variety of disciplines. In this chapter we are introducing a version of cognitive mapping which has been specifically developed to help internal and external consultants/facilitators deal with some important aspects of their job. [It] is founded on the belief . . . that language is a basic currency of organizational problem solving. When managers talk about an issue, and what should be done, they use language which is designed to argue why the world is 'like it is and how it might be changed'.

Take a simple example of one person expressing a view about profit sharing:

> The latter-day Labour Party, aiming to appeal upmarket, is in a more ambivalent position. At a time when they are looking for a concordat with the unions, union opposition to profit sharing – because of the fear of collective bargaining – is hard to avoid. American experience with Employee Share Ownership Plans since the early 1980s has led to a drop in union membership in firms with these profit sharing schemes.
>
> (McLoughlin 1986)

Figure 3.1 shows how this piece of written, rather than spoken, argument may be converted into a cognitive map. Important phrases are selected to capture the essential aspects of the arguments. An attempt to capture the meaning of each phrase is made by trying to identify the contrasting idea. Thus 'Labour support for profit sharing' is contrasted with 'ambivalence towards profit sharing', and 'upmarket appeal' is contrasted with 'working-class appeal'. This latter contrast is a possibly incorrect attempt by the coder to understand the meaning of 'upmarket' by making a guess . . . The meaning of a concept is given by the contrasting pole as well as the explanatory and consequential concepts; not by any dictionary definition.

The phrases and linking arrows are not precisely a replication of the language used by the person speaking: they have been modified to reflect the need for an action, or problem solving, orientation. Each of the concepts in Figure 3.1 is written as a 'call to action' and is intended to suggest an option for changing the nature of the situation in a positive way. Similarly, the argumentation (direction of the arrows) is such that an option always leads to a desired outcome, with the most important outcome hierarchically superior to others. The means to an end is always the subordinate concept, and placed at the tail of the arrow linking two concepts. In Figure 3.1 the highest order goal is taken to be the 'Labour Party seeking an upmarket appeal', alongside the other presumed goal of 'retaining Labour's concordat with the unions'. All the options are taken to have implications for these goals. In addition, the map indicates the nature of the argumentation by adding a negative sign to the end of an arrow if the first phrase of one concept relates to the second phrase of the other concept.

Early in a project it is important to build a map that reflects the client's, and no one else's, orientation to the problem (and particularly not that of the consultant).

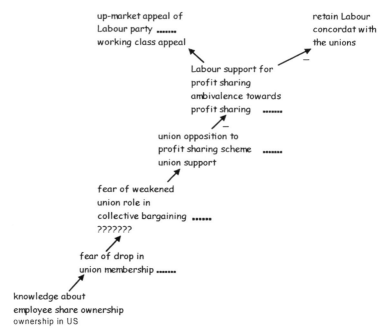

**Figure 3.1** An example of a small cognitive map

Note: . . . is read as 'rather than' and separates the first pole of the concept from the contrasting pole
Source: Eden and Ackerman (2001).

Changing the language used by the client, so that it becomes oriented to action rather than problem description, without the client losing 'ownership' of the model, is not a trivial exercise. Equally, deciding which concept is the goal/outcome/end and which is the action/option/means of a linked pair of concepts is an important part of the model building. For example, 'looking for a concordat with the unions' sounds like a goal (particularly given the use of the phrase 'looking for'), and so has been coded as a goal in Figure 3.1. However, if we were able to converse with Jane McLoughlin . . . we would be keen to establish whether 'a concordat' is regarded as a goal (a good outcome in its own right), or as an option which contributes to 'ambivalence towards profit sharing'. The overall sense of the text on its own makes us feel uncertain about our coding.

*Working with cognitive maps*

There are two principal ways of working on a map with the client. The first is to explore the goal system further, and then gradually work down the map towards increasingly detailed options for achieving goals. Alternatively, one can start from the detailed options and gradually work up the map towards goals by exploring each concept in turn as a potential option. Which of these two approaches is chosen depends upon the professional judgement of the consultant about process issues concerning client attitudes.

One of the powerful attributes of mapping as a model building method comes from the ability to create the model as the client is talking. This makes it possible to explore the implications of the model, with the client, during the interview. The consultant checks possible misunderstandings as the interview unfolds. This way of working also ensures that the consultant develops the questions asked during the interview from the interview data itself – rather than from a tight agenda of prepared questions. This allows for a warmer, more trusting consultant–client relationship to grow, and more importantly gives the control of the interview over to the client.

This style of operating allows the consultant to move in a gentle fashion from an 'empathetic' to a 'negotiative' paradigm of consultant–client relationship (Eden and Sims 1979). Early in the project the consultant must attend to understanding the world of the client from the client's perspective; later, and after trust has grown, the consultant can suggest alternative views. These alternative views may be based upon those of the consultant's substantive and content-related expertise from working on other similar projects, or can be based on injecting views from others in the problem solving group (but without identifying sources).

Working in the first mode, with the goal system, implies concentrating on the concepts at the 'top' part of the map. In our example this means concentrating on questions such as 'why is up-market appeal important to the Labour Party?' The client is invited to expand the chain of goals by moving to successively higher levels in the hierarchy. In this case we may suppose that something like 'wider electoral appeal . . . [to traditional supporters]' might be a further elaboration. Both client and consultant may find it illuminating to go on extending such questions until it becomes 'obvious' to both that the concept at the top of the model, with no further consequences, is 'self-evidently' a 'good thing'. Once this stage has been reached the client may be invited to work back gradually down the hierarchy by answering the question 'what options come to mind for changing this situation, other than those already mentioned?' For example, 'what other ways come to mind for shifting "ambivalence towards profit sharing" to "support", other than "reducing the fear of a weakened role in collective bargaining"?'

The second mode of working with the client focuses on action by identifying each 'tail' (the concept at the bottom of a chain of argumentation, that is with no further explanations) and testing it as a possible intervention point. Therefore, 'knowledge about share ownership in the United States' is tested as a possible option – is there any way in which this 'first pole' of the concept creatively suggests a 'contrasting pole'? It may seem more natural to regard this particular concept in the example as simply a part of the context within the original statement, rather than as a means to the end of 'reducing fear of a drop in union membership'. However, consideration of such concepts as potential options often leads to creative suggestions for action. In this case 'rubbishing the knowledge from the United States' might be such an option. The next part of the problem solving process is to consider other means by which it might be possible to reduce the 'fear of a drop in union membership'. So, we proceed to elaborate the map by inserting new options/tails as subordinate concepts to that being considered.

Further exploration of options moves up the concept hierarchy, by considering ways of making 'weakened role' an option. This is done in the same way as in the above example: in this case we had supposed that there was an action which might be taken to 'reduce the fear of a weakened role for collective bargaining', and had inserted '???' in Figure 3.1. This was to serve as a prompt for guiding the client to consider possible contrasting poles. In addition we would invite the client to consider other ways of 'reducing fear', by asking 'are there any other reasons why unions have a fear of weakened role of collective bargaining?'. After working with the client on other ways of countering weakened role by developing other new 'tails', we would then move to the next concept up the hierarchy and consider other ways of countering union opposition. And so on, elaborating the map by seeking to discover further explanations for why the situation is as it is.

Looking for options in this way reveals the importance of trying to identify contrasting poles of concepts – for the contrast is the essence of action. Each contrast has significantly different implications for identifying possible interventions and further explanations. Each explanation, in its own way, becomes a new option to be considered.

 **Activity 3.1**

Cognitive mapping is a technique for visualizing the way someone is thinking about a given topic in the form of a map. The map is thus a kind of explicit model of someone's conceptualization. What are the rules given by Eden and Ackerman for drawing maps of this kind?

 **Feedback**

The five rules for drawing up a cognitive map are:

1 Maps start by convention at the lower edge of the paper and work upwards.

2 Concepts should be written as calls to action, taking clients' concepts as the lead.

3 Concepts versus opposites are represented by dotted lines (. . . ) and should be read as 'rather than'.

4 Cause–effect relationships are represented by an arrow: (option → outcome).

5 A logic switch is indicated by a minus sign against an arrow-head (e.g. union opposition to profit-sharing scheme → – Labour support for profit-sharing).

The next extract from Eden and Ackermann explains the creation of a strategic map.

 **The strategic map**

Figure 3.1 is a 'cognitive' map because it is supposed to be a model of the thinking of one person. In a SODA project the cognitive map of each member of the client team will be merged to form an aggregated map called a 'strategic map'. The aim is to produce a 'facilitative device' to promote psychological negotiation amongst team members so that, in the first instance, a definition of the problem can be established. During the initial model building with individual clients, the aim was to help them 'change their minds' about the nature of the problem through a combination of self-reflection with respect to the map, and gentle negotiation with the consultant. The map is used as the device to facilitate the negotiation.

Similarly, the initial purpose of the merged map is to change the minds of each member of the client group, without their feeling compromised. The aim is to secure enough agreement about the nature of the problem that each team member is committed to expending energy on finding a portfolio of actions, where that portfolio is the strategy for dealing with the issue. The group negotiation approach is informed by some approaches to international conciliation, where the intention is to gain agreement to enough group ownership of the problem definition (the group map) and then move towards using the map as a way of encouraging the development of new options (or portfolios/systems of options) on which politically feasible agreement can be reached, rather than fighting over 'old options' (Fisher and Brown 1988).

Because the aim is to facilitate negotiation, the individual maps are merged with a significant regard for the anticipated dynamics of negotiation. This means that when a concept on one map is overlaid on a similar concept on another map, it is a matter of concern as to which person's wording is retained on the strategic map. Similarly, as the strategic map is analysed prior to creating an agenda for a SODA workshop, to be attended by all or most team members, then the extracts from the strategic map that are to be used in the workshop are carefully monitored to ensure balanced representation from key team members.

Consider the (unlikely) possibility that Jane McLoughlin is a member of a problem solving team and that one of her colleagues had said:

> It is possible that the Labour Party might support profit sharing schemes if opinion polls demonstrated support from Union members . . . however, the tabloid newspapers would need to give some education on profit sharing instead of continuing to ignore the idea . . . with support from these newspapers it is likely that some popular support might result – at the moment there is support only from the middle classes . . . it is also important that the 'man-in-the-street' is made aware of the benefits US workers have seen from profit sharing schemes in the US . . . the trouble for the Labour Party is that if there were popular support then other opposition parties might also support profit sharing . . . nevertheless I believe the crucial question for the Labour Party is whether their support could decrease antagonism from key [leaders of the business community] . . . I suspect that if there were mechanisms for applying profit sharing to public sector workers then this would be a powerful argument for the party supporting something which at present only seems to apply to the private sector.

These views could be shown as the map on the right of Figure 3.2, and the two maps merged along the following lines. We might overlay the two concepts that relate to profit sharing (concepts 1 and 5 in Figure 3.2), and then link concepts elsewhere within the two maps (4 leads to 2, 6 leads to 9, and 14 leads to 12 and 13). Unless there is a process reason for doing otherwise (for example, if the concept that is to be overlaid belongs to the boss, then it might be worth considering deliberately retaining it regardless of other considerations), then the concept that is lost is that which is less rich. Thus in this example concept 5 will be lost in favour of concept 1 which has a contrasting pole. As other concepts are linked, the consultant uses his judgement to maintain the hierarchical relationships within the final merged map. This judgement is not to be treated lightly, for the consultant will be beginning a process of negotiating his own view of the problem on to the model by inserting new links between 'owned' maps. For example, in the merged model, we have decided to suggest that a decrease in antagonism from key leaders [of the business community] will have the likely consequence of creating upmarket appeal. By so doing we are implicitly (and later during a workshop explicitly) inviting consideration of options for decreasing antagonism other than that of providing support for profit sharing.

Figure 3.2 shows instances of two paths of argumentation from one concept to another. For example, in the merged map concept 1 leads directly to concept 2 and indirectly through concept 4. In these circumstances it is helpful to ask whether there are genuinely two paths – it is often possible that the direct route is the same as the indirect route, the indirect route being a useful elaboration of the direct route. If the two paths indicate different argumentation – as appears to be the case in the map below – then it will be useful

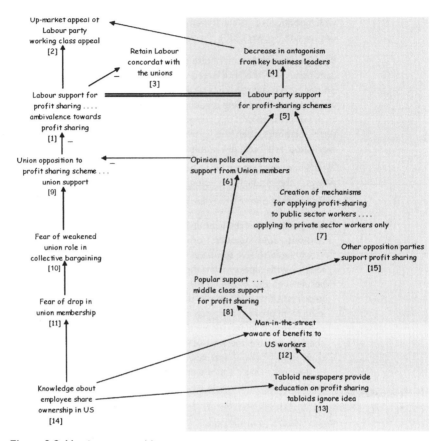

**Figure 3.2** Merging two cognitive maps
Notes:
1. Double lines connect similar concepts
2. Dotted lines show new relationships between concepts from different original maps
Source: Eden and Ackerman (2001).

to add in at least one further concept to explain the different means to the same end. In the example we might ask the clients to elaborate, and this might result in a further concept such as 'Labour seen to be supporting trendy new ideas'. We may also note that there are now ten (!) paths of argumentation from concept 14 to concept 2 (a path is any unique sequence of concepts, for example the path 14, 13, 12, 8, 6, 1, 2 is different from 14, 12, 8, 6, 1, 2). The option represented by concept 14 of rubbishing knowledge is a dilemma in that it leads to a desirable outcome following some paths and an undesirable outcome following others. It is also tempting for the consultant to insert a tentative negative link from the current undesirable negative-outcome of 'other opposition parties support profit sharing' to the goal of 'upmarket appeal'.

After maps have been merged, the consultant must analyse the content and structure of the model in order to generate an agenda for the workshop . . . The initial task is to analyse the data to identify 'emerging themes' (bundles or clusters of material that are tightly linked nodes), and 'core concepts' (those nodes, that if deleted, would fundamentally change the structure of the model).

*The workshop*

Typically, a workshop will be arranged to take anything from two hours to two days, depending on the availability of team members and the perceived importance of the issue. The scheme for the workshop is, in principle, similar to that for the interaction between consultant and single client. The consultant may choose to start from a goal orientation or an action orientation. An important consideration is to design an agenda which will allow a cyclic process to unfold. The objective of working with a cyclic process is to ensure that participants in a workshop are helped with the process of gradually absorbing the overall emerging issues, yet get to grips with the detail, and then move to action.

The aim of the first pass is to begin the process of participants 'taking on board' alternative views – the gradual psychological negotiation of a new construction of the problem, and ownership by enough of the group view for negotiation to occur. The first pass contributes to gaining this ownership by a controlled 'walk' through the model to demonstrate that concepts belonging to each participant have been included in the model. The potential for each of the participants 'changing his or her mind' is largely dependent upon the help the model provides in extending ownership beyond those concepts that belong to a single participant. Extending ownership occurs by a participant seeing his or her own concepts now set within the context of concepts that are known to belong to other participants.

The first pass creates a 'backdrop' against which the second pass, focusing on individual issues/clusters, can unfold. The consultant must decide whether to work on a cluster top-down (goal system mode) or bottom-up (option mode). In this second pass the 'rules' change and discussion is encouraged.

 **Activity 3.2**

SODA uses a workshop format for problem structuring and strategy formation.

1  How might a typical workshop involve the facilitator and participants?
2  What would you add to your list of rules for cognitive mapping so as to cover strategic mapping as well?

 **Feedback**

1  A typical workshop would involve:

- recruiting participants and having a first discussion of the problem/situation
- an interview with each participant to identify their concepts and ideas about the problem. This may involve using a tape recorder
- transcribing the tapes into a provisional cognitive map for each individual
- holding a second interview to amend and confirm the map
- merging individual cognitive maps into a strategic map and running a group workshop which uses the strategic map as an agenda.

2  An additional rule might be 'Individual maps are merged to form a strategic map by choosing the richer of two similar formulations. Sometimes it will be necessary to keep both (e.g. where the contrasting poles represent different opposites), in which case an undirected line between the two can indicate the connection.'

## SODA in action

SODA has been used in a range of areas, including health services. As you will see in the following case study, there may be some variations in the standard format of the approach.

The following extract from a working paper by Gains and Rosenhead (1993) is about how they used SODA during the introduction of a hospital quality assurance programme. This will give you a better understanding of how SODA can be used in strategy formation.

###  Cognitive mapping in an English district hospital

At the time of the project, audit was a sensitive topic, and it was thought desirable to start by meeting key members of the group individually to explain the nature of the project and to answer any queries or doubts. (This additional stage would probably be unnecessary where the initiative for a project originated with the client group.) The agreement and commitment of the group were obtained, and all of the members agreed to participate in the mapping process. They included [ten] individuals in the categories of consultant, registrar, junior doctor, nurse, and manager.

The generation of ten individual cognitive maps is a considerable undertaking. At one point, the joint mapping of three junior doctors as a group was considered, as a means of reducing this load. In the end it was decided to proceed on an individual basis, and it did indeed prove that they had distinctively different contributions to make. Evidently choices of this kind present a tension between economy and comprehensiveness which needs to be considered in the light of specific circumstances.

As the project team were inexperienced in the substantive content of audit, it was decided to hold all interview sessions with two team members participating, rather than a single interviewer as is normal. Using just one interviewer has the advantage of economising on the use of human resources, and runs less risk of intimidating the interviewee. However, the advantage of involving two team members is the reduced risk of missing concepts, links or points to probe further during the interview.

After each interview, the project team incorporated any revisions into the individual's map. This was then prepared in a well-structured and easy-to-read form, both for the individual to retain, and to assist the process of merging the various maps.

*The strategic workshop*

The strategic workshop was held at one of the monthly paediatric audit meetings. Only six of the ten members who had contributed maps were present; others had conflicting commitments or had changed posts. Three new members of the paediatric group also attended, and the Regional Audit Coordinator was present for part of the proceedings. Necessarily the discussion which took place, like the map which stimulated it, was specific to the particular group whose views it represented. Nevertheless that discussion will be summarised here as part of the evidence on which any provisional assessment of the method's more general utility can be based.

The meeting was opened by the senior member of the project team acting as facilitator, who led the group through the structure of the merged map. This was done at first in broad terms only, indicating the major sectors of audit activity which seemed to emerge from the elicited concepts and linking relationships.

In discussion a group member observed that this structure was incomplete, and that a further, monitoring activity was required. This was generally agreed by those at the meeting, who felt that the Audit Office could have a valuable role in monitoring the effects of changes in practice, once agreed. It should be noted that the monitoring activity had not been present in any of the individual cognitive maps, but was elicited by the attempt in discussion to structure and make sense of their joint perceptions as represented in the merged map.

The result seemed to be the generation of group 'ownership' of the necessity of monitoring, which was seen as an inherent part of the activity which they were engaged in, rather than a bureaucratic imposition. And, indeed, this acceptance led to an 'in principle' agreement on what was seen as an appropriate consequential activity by the Audit Office.

*The map in more detail*

Attention was then turned to the more detailed structure of the merged map. Given the time limitation, the discussion was encouraged by the facilitator to range freely over the map, with a view to identifying areas of interest to the group; no attempt was made to achieve systematic coverage of all areas, which would only have ensured a uniformly superficial treatment.

One issue discussed at some length was that of inappropriate referrals from the Casualty department. The high referral rate was thought to be due to a combination of two factors: the lack of feedback to Casualty on what were felt by paediatricians to be inappropriate referrals, and the fact that junior doctors in Casualty were (due to the dynamics of the medical career system) often the most inexperienced in the hospital. The focus of the discussion then shifted to the understandable reasons why on occasions inappropriate referrals might occur – due for example, to media and time pressures.

It was agreed that if the issue persisted, then representatives from Casualty should be invited to discuss it at an audit meeting. One idea canvassed was that progress might be made by a smaller group using the mapping technique to explore that pathway in more detail, for further consideration at the full audit meeting. This more focused approach, it was thought, might have application in other areas of concern also.

*Future audit practice*

This audit meeting was regarded by all participants as principally one to assess the output of the mapping process. Therefore most discussion was conducted in an exploratory mode, with no prior assumption that decisions should result.

However, some firmer commitments about the future practice of audit were arrived at. One was that letters of complaint received should be treated as high priority for audit discussion – interestingly, a method of getting topics onto the audit agenda which none of the ten individual maps had incorporated. It was proposed by a junior doctor during the 'taking stock' period towards the end of the meeting, and was received positively.

Another decision was that the following month's audit meeting should be on a topic selected by, and run by, junior doctors. There was considerable enthusiasm to get on with the concrete practice of audit. It was proposed by the audit group that further assistance from the project team (if available) should be deferred for at least a few months. It was thought likely that this would be most helpful after some 'normal' audit sessions had identified one or more priority areas which could benefit from more detailed attention.

Taking a longer perspective, it was proposed that there should be an annual plan for audit, which should ensure at least a sprinkling of 'tough' or 'uncomfortable' topics, including those which cognitive mapping had helped identify. What distinguished such topics was not articulated. The Audit Office as an identifiable unit for the foreseeable future was seen as preferable to the absorption of the administrative aspects of audit into the various clinical departments. Indeed, an expansion of its role was seen as desirable.

A particularly interesting proposal was to use the map as it developed as an 'organisational memory'. The paediatric group, in common with other specialties, has a high turnover particularly of more junior members. The map, it was suggested, could, if continuously updated, make the group's current thinking on audit readily accessible to new members. This proposal, generated spontaneously from the audit group, in fact mirrors discussion by practitioners of cognitive mapping.

*Feedback*

Immediately after the strategic map meeting participants were asked to fill in a short open-ended questionnaire. Though the (anonymous) responses are specific to the particular group and project they do indicate certain dimensions of reaction. The main features of this feedback are presented and discussed below.

Three of the eight attending participants initially found the mapping notation easy to grasp, but the others found it difficult. This may well have been because the verbally-based technique was 'alien' to them, the majority having a scientific, rather than a managerial, training. A non-quantitative modelling approach aimed at facilitating group interaction is far from the medical-scientific paradigm of investigation.

After the initial culture shock, however, six of the eight said that they found the process of developing their maps to be a positive one. Specific reasons offered for this were that the map was a useful and enjoyable focus, and that it was valuable to have ideas challenged. On the negative side, one participant found the purpose of the map unclear and another found it of no use. One possible contributory factor was that both of these participants found the notation difficult to grasp.

All but one of the attending participants found the group session to be beneficial as a team-building experience, an aid to decision making, and a focus for future plans. Positive aspects noted included the value of seeing differences and similarities in each others' ideas, and provision of an overview of ultimate goals.

Additional feedback was received from Dr. S as a member of the group who had been unable to attend the workshop session. Prior to her appointment as Acting Director of Public Health for the area, she had direct responsibility for promoting audit throughout the health authority. By comparison with other audit groups in the District, she found the paediatric group had a clearly steeper learning curve. From an initial situation of hesitancy and even disquiet, they had moved to commitment and purposeful activity in a markedly shorter time. It was particularly noticeable that junior staff, initially almost voiceless passengers, became much more active in their contributions. In any such process both group characteristics and methodology play a part. However, Dr. S's view was that the methodology employed had been a significant factor in the progress achieved.

**Activity 3.3**

Imagine that you had been involved in this study. Transcripts of three of the interviews, drawn up by Rosenhead, are provided below:

- a junior doctor's interview. (Among the junior doctor's concerns is the additional workload arising from audit.)
- a consultant's (senior doctor's) interview. (This doctor hopes to achieve better care through protocols based on audit.)
- a manager's interview. (The manager is hoping to get better contracts if audit is implemented.)

Choose one of the transcripts, examine its content, and draw a cognitive map for it using the five rules listed in the feedback to Activity 3.1.

 **Transcripts**

*The junior doctor's interview*

One of the problems of audit from my perspective is that it's yet another job we have to take on. It's quite crucial that there should be good support from the Audit Office, so that it isn't down to junior doctors to do the dogsbody work, as usual. If we have to spend even more time, extracting material from case notes for example, we'll end up doing even more overtime. As it is, most of the time we're too tired to learn – so how are we going to get a decent postgraduate education? But if audit isn't educational, I don't see how it can be judged a success.

I suppose that one good thing about audit is that, if the audit meetings work properly, we do get exposed to more than one point of view, and that's a good feature for a postgraduate education. The audit meeting can critically evaluate our practice – but only if people feel free to speak. That is certainly much easier if cases are considered confidentially, that is, without everything being traced back to whoever may not have done things quite right. One thing that can make it hard to speak is if some people at the meeting have personalities that don't lend themselves to group working. And of course, if there is competition between the consultants, so that they start disagreeing with each other, then there is little chance of the audit meeting being constructive.

What have I forgotten to mention? Oh yes, in some areas our case notes really aren't up to scratch. Getting that right would certainly help audit meetings along. And if we had improved case notes, that would be a good step towards improving our practice. Something our consultants could do is to take up the issues that surface at audit meetings with other departments. Often the improvements that are needed are out there, not in our own department. For example, we need to reduce the incidence of inappropriate referrals from Casualty. Improving our practice would certainly improve morale in the group, and that in itself would help to make audit a success.

*The manager's interview*

As I see it, audit (so long as it is carried out properly and thoroughly) has a lot to offer to the practice of medical care in this hospital. For one thing, it can enable us to establish reasonable standards of care that can be the basis of contracts with purchasers. If we've got some numbers and protocols for more of the standard conditions, then my job in fixing quality standards which we can attach to contracts with some confidence would be much easier. Not all purchasers are that interested in quality, but some do demand quality, and if we haven't got quantitative standards, it can be a tricky business. So you could say that if it helps us to get contracts, then audit is a success for us. If we can get enough good contracts, we can use the resources to provide a better quality of care.

Of course, that's not the only advantage. For one thing, the audit meeting is one place where junior doctors can challenge the consultants. Beliefs can be challenged, and it avoids tunnel vision. So that makes audit an educational process all round, and that can only be a benefit.

What we've got to do is make sure that enough resources are put into the audit function. Clerical support from the audit office is crucial – preparing agendas, making sure everyone gets reminders of the meeting time, that sort of thing. Without that, many of the staff would simply fail to show up – especially the consultants! And without enough of the staff there, there is no way you are going to get a productive audit meeting.

One spin-off from audit is that when the group finds something which could be done better, or at least more consistently, then it's a real benefit as far as training is concerned. It gives us a real fix on training needs, and we can make sure that the gap is plugged. That's true for both nurses and junior doctors. It's never too late to learn!

*The senior doctor's interview*

The only criterion of whether audit is a success is whether better care is given – that is, whether patients actually experience better outcomes. Needless to say, we can only do that if we are also given the resources, which depends on getting decent contracts.

We mustn't forget, either, that many staff in the department are just passing through on their way to other jobs in the health service. We need to make sure that for them audit is a learning experience. And I don't just mean doctors, but nurses as well. One good result of our audit meetings for them will be if we can make care plans more effective. That's one of the best ways for them to learn.

Certainly a well-prepared and well-run audit meeting can greatly improve communication between staff, and so lead to greater openness. That would be a bonus for group morale.

One of my biggest hopes from audit is that we will be able to establish more and better protocols. That really needs the impetus of a discussion at an audit meeting behind it, so that people will understand the priority. Well thought-out protocols can usefully be included in contracts – and it will help us to get them.

A spin-off of audit is that we should get better outcome measures. Finding out how well we are doing should help us to do better. We must be careful, of course. If audit is going to be used to set standards, we must make sure that they are realistic. They must take all circumstances into account.

⟲ **Feedback**

You should compare your map with the relevant one from Figures 3.3 to 3.5. Note that each cognitive map is an attempt to capture the language used by the client.

The strategic map combining all individual maps is shown in Figure 3.6, providing a conceptual framework for structuring audit as a self-managed process in a hospital setting.

It can be seen that in this case the strategic map has involved simplification. Some of the intermediate links (such as 'junior doctors do more overtime') have been dropped. Some of the similar concepts from different maps have been taken as equivalent. Examples are 'improve practice' with 'give better care' and 'expose junior doctors to more than one view' with 'beliefs are challenged'.

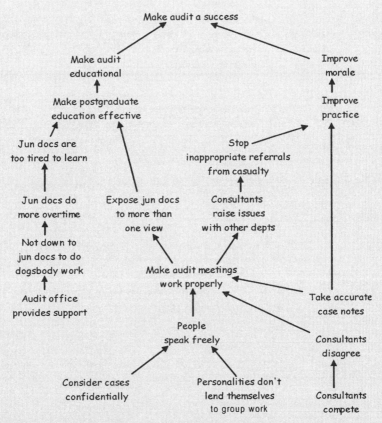

**Figure 3.3** The junior doctor's cognitive map

Source: Adapted from Rosenhead and Mingers (2001).

On this basis a number of 'firmer' commitments were made, including ways of choosing items for the audit agenda; confirming and expanding the role of the audit office rather than absorbing its functions into different clinical departments; and using the map to explain the approach to audit to new hospital staff.

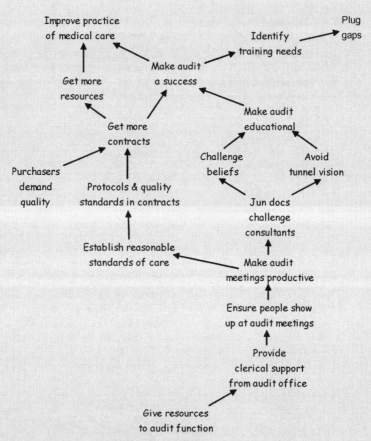

**Figure 3.4** The manager's cognitive map

Source: Adapted from Rosenhead and Mingers (2001).

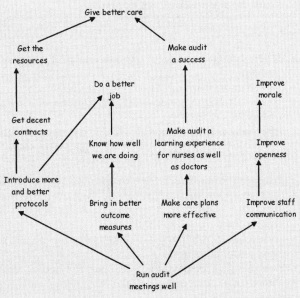

**Figure 3.5** The senior doctor's cognitive map

Source: Adapted from Rosenhead and Mingers (2001).

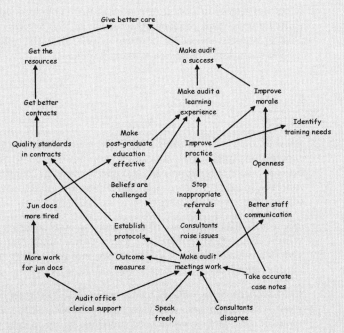

**Figure 3.6** The strategic map combining individual maps

Source: Adapted from Rosenhead and Mingers (2001).

## Potential strengths and weaknesses of the approach

In summary:

- SODA brings a range of perspectives and expertise to understanding the problem.
- Shared understanding helps build commitment.
- Understanding may help with real conflicts of interest and dissolve apparent ones.
- Maps may help communicate ideas to others outside the original process.

Arguably, potential problems with using SODA in a health care context are:

- It takes time and money, so is best for big/one-off problems.
- It needs a competent facilitator and these are in short supply.
- It is hard to select a manageable number (about 10) when there are many stakeholders.
- It depends on willingness to participate and concern for wider objectives than strict personal interest.
- It may expose latent conflicts and may not help in resolving them.
- Professional and organizational hierarchies, common in health care, can impede the process.
- It may be manipulated by powerful or adept stakeholders.
- The step from shared understanding to shared commitment to action is a large one.
- It is a qualitative technique and so cannot help directly with questions of 'how much'.

In the context of this book, it is important to conclude this list of pros and cons with the point that problem structuring, as well as being valuable in itself, can provide a relatively secure basis on which to start building more quantitative models of the kinds described in later chapters.

## Summary

SODA is based on a psychological theory that people continually strive to make sense of their world through trial and error. Their perceptions influence their expectations and their expectations influence their perceptions. The medium through which this happens is the construct system. People's constructs are used to conceive, manage and control the outside world. Individual construct systems may adapt and change over time.

In line with this theory, an organization is seen as a setting of changing coalitions of individuals who negotiate their views. Politics and power play an important role in decision making. The SODA approach builds explicitly on negotiation to solve complex problems.

SODA recognizes the value of teamwork in strategy formation. Organizations build teams because synergies add value over and above the sum of each individual's contributions. The experiences of individual team members can make a valuable contribution to decision making.

The key technique of SODA is cognitive mapping. A cognitive map provides a visual representation (a graphic model) of an individual's or group's concepts. This model is amenable to formal analysis. SODA needs a facilitator to manage consensus. Much depends on the ability and experience of the facilitator to achieve commitment to the approach.

## References

Buzan T with Buzan B (1993) *The Mind Map Book*. London: BBC Books.

Eden C (1988) Cognitive mapping: a review. *European Journal of Operational Research* 36: 1–13.

Eden C and Ackerman F (2001) SODA – the principles, in J. Rosenhead and J. Mingers (eds) *Rational Analysis for a Problematic World Revisited*, pp. 21–41. Chichester: John Wiley & Sons.

Eden C and Sims D (1979) On the nature of problems in consulting practice. *Omega* 7: 119–27.

Eden C, Ackermann F and Cropper S (1992) The analysis of cause maps. *Journal of Management Studies* 29: 309–24.

Fisher R and Brown S (1988) *Getting Together: Building a Relationship that Gets to Tes*. Boston: Houghton-Mifflin.

Gains A and Rosenhead J (1993) *Problem Structuring for Medical Quality Assurance*. Working paper No. LSEOR 93.8. London: LSE.

Kelly GA (1955) *The Psychology of Personal Constructs*. New York: WW Norton.

McLoughlin J (1986) Who gains from profit-sharing? *The Guardian*, 14 May.

Quinn JB (1980) *Strategies/or Change: Logical Incrementalism*. Homewood, IL: Irwin.

Rosenhead J and Mingers J (eds) (2001) *Rational Analysis for a Problematic World Revisited*. Chichester: John Wiley & Sons.

Silverman D (1970) *The Theory of Organizations*. London: Heinemann.

Tolman EC (1948) Cognitive maps in rats and men. *Psychological Review* 55: 189–208.

# SECTION 2

# Methods for clarifying complex decisions

# 4 | Many criteria

This chapter and the next two introduce some of the methods that can help in structuring and clarifying complex decisions. There are few circumstances is which it is possible to identify a solution as unequivocally the best one. In this chapter you will learn about methods that can help when there are many, usually conflicting, criteria. You will take the first steps towards structuring a decision problem by developing sets of criteria and options. You will then be given the performance ratings of a set of options and will try a variety of methods of shortlisting, ranking and choosing 'good' options.

It is often impossible to be sure, at the time that the decision has to be made, which course of action will lead to a desired outcome. In Chapter 5 you will look more closely at ways of dealing with uncertainty about the future, about values and about the boundaries of the decision problem. In Chapter 6 you will consider a 'risk'-based approach, which depends on estimates of the probabilities of different hypothetical 'futures' becoming reality.

## Learning objectives

**By the end of this chapter, you will be better able to:**

- **identify and clarify the decision options and criteria in a decision making problem**
- **describe three approaches (weighting, satisficing and sequential elimination) to decision making with multiple criteria**
- **understand one approach to calculating weights for criteria based on pairwise preferences**

## Key terms

**Decision criteria** Characteristics used in judgements about preferences, or measures of performance, against which decision options are assessed. They usually relate to benefits or achievement of objectives; to cost or risks; and to feasibility.

**Dominated option** A decision option that may be similar to another option in terms of some criteria but is inferior to it in others.

## Why rational decision making is difficult

In Chapter 1 you learned that 'substantive' rationality was difficult in health care decision making.

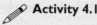 **Activity 4.1**

What were some of the difficulties identified?

 **Feedback**

- There may be many criteria because decision makers generally have many objectives.
- Different decision makers and stakeholders may be uncertain or disagree about the ratings of particular options, or the importance or weight that they attach to each criterion.
- Factors beyond the knowledge or control of the decision makers may influence how well a particular course of action actually 'performs', so that the outcome of a particular decision will be difficult to predict.
- There may be so many potential options and criteria that the decision makers suffer from information overload and need help in taking so many factors into account.

You will now learn about some methods that can help with these types of difficulty. In this chapter, the focus will be on dealing with multiple criteria.

## One criterion vs many

In Chapter 2 you designed and analysed a simple health care programme. Apart from only involving three diseases, as a decision problem it was simplified structurally in three important ways:

- For all except the final task there was *only one criterion*: to maximize the number of premature deaths avoided for a given budget.
- The number of premature deaths avoided depended primarily on *your decision*; other factors were assumed to be constant over the time period of interest.
- While there was some *uncertainty* about the impact of different levels of expenditure because of concerns over the accuracy of the information provided, the uncertain values were expected to fall within a given range, and so the implications of the uncertainty could be explored using sensitivity analysis.

Decision analysts describe this kind of decision as a *single criterion problem*. The key point was made at the end of Chapter 2: this is the only type of problem for which you can be sure that there is an unequivocal best or *optimum* solution. Where there is more than one criterion, the decision that is best in terms of one criterion may not be best in terms of others, and different decision makers and stakeholders may disagree about what is important.

It is quite common to see magazine articles aimed at helping people choose something like a car or a washing machine. If these articles are well researched, they may include a table. Usually this will have the possible options listed down the side and criteria such as cost, performance, reliability, style and safety across the top. In each 'cell' in the table there will be an indication of how well one of the options (rows in the table) performs in terms of one of the criteria (columns). This may take the form of a number, or a category on a scale from very good to very bad, or possibly a reference to text in a footnote. This kind of attempt to set out the pros and cons of each option in a systematic way has a long history. Here is a celebrated letter from Benjamin Franklin to Joseph Priestley:

 **Letter to Joseph Priestley**

London, 19 September 1772

Dear Sir

In the Affair of so much Importance to you, wherein you ask my Advice, I cannot, for want of sufficient Premises, advise you what to determine, but if you please I will tell you how. When those difficult Cases occur, they are difficult, chiefly because while we have them under Consideration, all the Reasons pro and con are not present to the Mind at the same time; but sometimes one Set present themselves, and at other times another, the first being out of sight. Hence the various Purposes or Inclinations that alternately prevail, and the Uncertainty that perplexes us. To get over this, my Way is to divide half a Sheet of Paper by a Line into two Columns; writing over the one Pro, and over the other Con. Then, during three or four Days Consideration, I put down under the different Heads short Hints of the different Motives, that at different Times occur to me, for or against the Measure. When I have thus got them all together in one View, I endeavor to estimate their respective Weights; and where I find two, one on each side, that seem equal, I strike them both out. If I find a Reason pro equal to some two Reasons con, I strike out the three. If I judge some two Reasons con, equal to some three Reasons pro, I strike out the five; and thus proceeding I find at length where the Balance lies; and if, after a Day or two of further Consideration, nothing new that is of importance occurs on either Side, I come to a Determination accordingly. And, tho' the Weight of Reasons cannot be taken with the Precision of algebraic Quantities, yet when each is thus considered, separately and comparatively, and the whole lies before me, I think I can judge better, and am less liable to make a rash Step, and in fact I have found great Advantage from this kind of equation, in what may be called Moral or Prudential Algebra.

Wishing sincerely that you may determine for the best, I am ever, my dear Friend, Yours most affectionately.

B Franklin

This letter captures both the motivation for and some of the elements of multiple criteria decision analysis. The idea is to provide help in the form of how, rather than what, to decide; and this involves identification of the options (in this case given); reflection on what should be taken into account in the comparison; assembly of the necessary information and its presentation in digestible form; and a process for arriving at a choice.

In many cases the methodological contribution of the analyst stops once the relevant information has been identified, assembled and presented. Figure 4.1 is an example of a comparative advantage chart for two approaches to developing

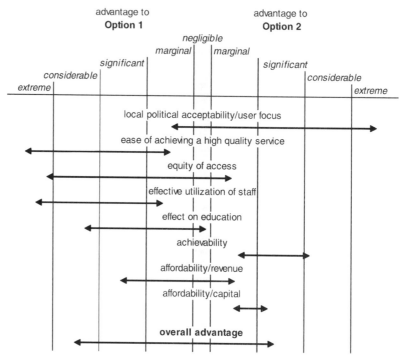

**Figure 4.1** Comparative advantage chart for two schemes for children's services
Source: Cushman and Rosenhead (2004).

children's health services. Option 1 involved a single in-patient unit and a large increase in community provision, and Option 2 involved two in-patient units and a moderate increase in community provision. For each option and criterion it shows a range of possible values, indicating an element of uncertainty in the assessment. This particular way of capturing and presenting the data is part of a broader approach to strategic planning called Strategic Choice (Friend and Hickling 2004) to which you will return in Chapter 5. There are many variations in the design of such visual aids.

In this case production of the chart was a sufficient basis for the stakeholders to agree on Option 1. (The more politically charged issue of where to site the single unit was considered separately!) In other situations, where there are many more options, further analysis may be required.

## The performance matrix or consequence table

For most multiple criteria problems the construction of the framework of options and criteria, in the form of a grid or table, is a useful first step towards identifying the information needed to make a decision. Completing the table provides a way of organizing and presenting the information.

The essential activities are as follows:

1 *Identify the decision context.* What is the overall aim of the organization? And who is involved or affected? Roy (1996) distinguishes between stakeholders who have 'an important interest in the decision and will intervene to directly affect it through [their] value systems' and third parties 'who do not actively participate in the decision, but who are affected by its consequences and whose preferences must be considered when arriving at the decision'.

2 *Develop a set of criteria.* Criteria and objectives are very closely related, so one good starting point is to list your objectives and see how they can be turned into criteria. For example, an objective might be open-ended (reduce a readmission rate) or specific (reduce a readmission rate by 10 per cent). In both cases, the criterion is the readmission rate. If you are unclear about your objectives, brainstorming may help; this involves intensive, more or less structured discussion among decision makers to generate ideas, perhaps by exploring what would distinguish a good option from a bad one.

3 *Identify the decision options.* This may again be a matter of brainstorming but problem structuring methods may be helpful.

4 *Devise measurement scales or scoring systems for each criterion.* These scales will depend on the data available, the significance of the decision, and the time and resources available for data collection. The ratings might be based on subjective judgements, on direct observation and data analysis, or on estimates derived by using a model.

5 *Rate the options* according to the measurement scales.

You may need to repeat these steps until a satisfactory framework is achieved. Also the ordering of tasks 2 and 3 is reversed in some cases. For example, the options may be determined for you. In this case one possible approach to generating criteria is as follows:

1 List the advantages and disadvantages of Option 1 compared to the existing situation.

2 For each advantage or disadvantage, identify a corresponding criterion (a variable, not an attribute, e.g. 'cost', not 'cheap').

3 List the advantages and disadvantages of Option 2 compared to the existing arrangement and Option 1.

4 Add to the list of criteria if need be.

5 Continue with the other options until no new criteria arise.

6 Finally, shorten the list of criteria by removing any which essentially measure the same thing (it being important to avoid double-counting) or which do not discriminate (i.e. according to which all the options are similar).

Any formal analysis of the performance matrix that may follow will be a great deal easier if the criteria are 'preference independent', i.e. there should be no additional advantage or disadvantage in particular *combinations* of ratings. For example, if a meal made up of your favourite dishes is not your favourite meal, your gastronomic judgement involves preference dependence.

One common difficulty is that the objectives and/or criteria may be abstractions and so cannot be measured directly. Examples include 'the health of the population', 'quality of care' or the 'organization's prospect of survival'. In this situation the simple approach is to rate the options by making explicit judgements (e.g.

rating the impact of the option as good, fair or poor). Otherwise you have to oper-
ationalize the abstraction by choosing one or more indicators. Mortality rates are
often taken as indicators of a population's health, for example, and case fatality
rates as indicators of quality of care. Use of the word 'indicator' implies a recognition that your measurement and your criterion are not the same, and typically the
broader the abstraction, the larger the number of indicators needed to capture it
adequately.

In this situation it can be helpful to form a hierarchy or 'value tree' showing the
relationships between the various dimensions of the problem. Health has been
famously broken down into its physical, mental and social aspects. In older people
the physical dimension may be broken down into scores for pain and disability;
disability may be split into mobility, sight and hearing, and so forth. However, this
creates a new problem: how to present large amounts of data in ways that are
digestible but avoid controversial assumptions about the relative values of very
different kinds of benefit.

This kind of problem mainly occurs when rating benefits. Costs may also be organ-
ized in a hierarchy; accommodation costs may be split into one-off and recurring;
recurring costs split into rent, maintenance and utilities; utilities into water, elec-
tricity, etc. Here, though, there will be no problem with aggregation (adding the
different components together) if everything is measured in money terms in the
first place. The issue is whether you will need to keep some costs in separate categories if, for example, expenditure under different budget headings has different
implications.

 **Activity 4.2**

A decision has to be made about extending the main operating theatre block of
an acute hospital. Currently, the hospital has six theatres for in-patient surgery, with
capacity to perform 12,000 operations per year. The hospital managers believe that
there is unmet demand for this service and the potential to expand up to 16,000
operations per year. They are considering building another two theatres, each with a
capacity to perform 2000 operations per year.

In terms of Roy's definitions, who might be the stakeholders and who the third parties
in this decision?

 **Feedback**

As well as hospital managers, stakeholders are likely to include senior hospital staff and
representatives from funding organizations. They might also include representatives of:

• professional or staff groups
• patients
• neighbouring health care providers.

It might also include public health practitioners with a brief to represent the health
care needs of the wider population. How wide the net is spread will be a matter of
management style and custom.

**Activity 4.3**

What are the decision options? You should think beyond the obvious ones implied in the question.

 **Feedback**

Option generation could be the subject of a brainstorming session. One advantage of this is that other decision makers can suggest options that might not have occurred to you. The obvious options are:

- build 0, 1 or 2 theatres.

However, there are others such as:

- increase throughput in the current theatre block by improving efficiency, putting on additional shifts, etc.
- contract out some of the operations to other hospitals
- adopt different combinations of these two options.

This last point is worth emphasizing. In some decision problems (such as choice of a site for a health centre), the different options are essentially substitutes for one another. You can only build the health centre in one place. In other, generally more complex situations, the options can be complementary and the issue becomes what is the best mix of different types of option. This type of question is addressed in more depth in Chapter 8.

 **Activity 4.4**

What criteria would you use in deciding on which option to pursue?

 **Feedback**

One possible framework for developing a set of criteria is given in Table 4.1.

**Table 4.1** Criteria for selecting an option

| advantages/disadvantages/benefits/costs to *patients/ carers* | • effect on health/quality of life/satisfaction<br>• effect on distance travelled to service<br>• effect on waiting time for service<br>• effect on costs borne by patients/carers, etc. |
| --- | --- |
| advantages/disadvantages/costs/savings/other benefits to *payers/health system* | • one-off costs: buildings, equipment, training<br>• recurrent/revenue costs: staff, consumables, depreciation/maintenance, etc.<br>• income generation |

*Continued*

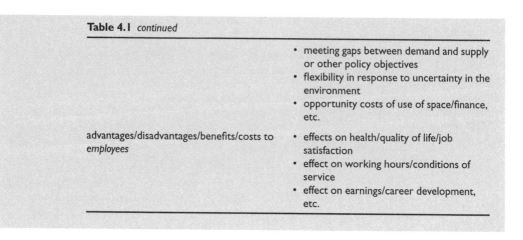

**Table 4.1** *continued*

| | |
|---|---|
| | • meeting gaps between demand and supply or other policy objectives |
| | • flexibility in response to uncertainty in the environment |
| | • opportunity costs of use of space/finance, etc. |
| advantages/disadvantages/benefits/costs to employees | • effects on health/quality of life/job satisfaction |
| | • effect on working hours/conditions of service |
| | • effect on earnings/career development, etc. |

## Analysing the performance matrix

Often the process of developing and filling in the performance matrix is sufficient as a basis for decision making but where there are many options and criteria it may still be difficult to see what to do. The following activity provides an example of this.

Table 4.2 is a performance matrix intended to help choose the location of a health centre. The decision makers have identified 20 possible sites and five criteria. For some of the criteria the options are rated qualitatively as poor; fair or good. For the

**Table 4.2** Which site for a health centre?

| Site | Staff acceptability | Accessibility for patients | Quality of environment | Running costs £k | Capital cost £k |
|---|---|---|---|---|---|
| 1 | good | fair | poor | 1700 | 3000 |
| 2 | fair | fair | good | 2300 | 3800 |
| 3 | poor | fair | fair | 2100 | 4200 |
| 4 | fair | good | fair | 1200 | 5200 |
| 5 | poor | fair | fair | 2100 | 1400 |
| 6 | good | good | good | 1800 | 3800 |
| 7 | good | poor | good | 800 | 4200 |
| 8 | fair | poor | fair | 700 | 5000 |
| 9 | fair | fair | fair | 1800 | 4000 |
| 10 | good | good | good | 1000 | 4800 |
| 11 | good | fair | good | 2100 | 3700 |
| 12 | fair | good | fair | 1100 | 5400 |
| 13 | poor | fair | fair | 1700 | 2000 |
| 14 | fair | good | good | 2500 | 4000 |
| 15 | poor | good | fair | 1800 | 2400 |
| 16 | poor | fair | poor | 2100 | 2000 |
| 17 | poor | good | good | 1600 | 1400 |
| 18 | fair | poor | good | 600 | 1900 |
| 19 | fair | poor | fair | 700 | 3400 |
| 20 | good | fair | fair | 1200 | 5000 |

running and capital cost criteria, estimates are provided in units of £1000. Given this information, how would you set about making a shortlist of options for more detailed investigation?

There are many approaches to this, but the three main categories of approach are:

1 *Satisficing*. It may be that there are a number of characteristics that every option must have if it is to be worth further consideration. For example, some options might, on discussion or preliminary investigation, turn out be unacceptable to staff, unsafe or well above budget. Satisficing involves setting standards for what is 'good enough' for each criterion and then eliminating any option that does not meet these standards. This method is commonly used in shortlisting candidates for a job. This may eliminate very few candidates – or all of them. In Table 4.2, if a 'poor' on any of the first three criteria made an option unacceptable, 11 options would be eliminated.

2 *Weighting*. First transform the ratings into scores, so that a higher score means 'more preferred' for each criterion. For example, the cost criteria in Table 4.2 would have to be reversed, so that higher scores are better. Then assign an importance 'weight' to each criterion. Multiply each score by the relevant weight, and add all the weighted scores for each option together (or average them) so as to give an *overall score* for each option. This is called *linear additive* weighting, the most straightforward way of combining scores and weights, and the one that many people think of first, although there are others.

Potentially this has advantages in terms of consistency of decision making (if A is preferred to B and B to C, A should be preferred to C). However, for a number of reasons it is difficult to use weighting methods appropriately:

(a) Scores have to be on equal-interval strength-of-preference scales; rankings are not good enough. What this means is that if ratings of poor, fair and good are to be transformed into scores of 0, 1 and 2, the amount by which fair is preferred to poor has to be the same as the amount by which good is preferred to fair.

(b) If different criteria are rated on different scales (lives saved, financial cost, etc.), this will have to be taken into account, either in the scores or in the criterion 'importance' weights. In this example, 'capital costs' start with more implicit weight than the other scales because the range of values in Table 4.2 is larger.

(c) Preference ratings on each criterion should be mutually independent, with no additional advantage or disadvantage in particular combinations of ratings.

Faced with all these requirements, how do you choose the weights? And what do you do if the decision makers disagree about what they should be? Arguments among decision makers about what option is best can easily turn into less grounded arguments about choosing whichever weights produce the answer they want. Weighting is a deceptively simple method that can be misleading and there is a strong case for trying less demanding methods first.

3 *Sequential elimination*. Option A is said to dominate Option B if it scores better than, or as well as, Option B on all criteria. If this is the case, you should be able to eliminate Option B without having made any value judgements. This has the attraction of being a relatively transparent and undemanding method. It only requires agreement about the broad ranking of each option on each

criterion. The relative importance of each *criterion* does not come into it, so it may allow uncontroversial simplification of a problem. It does have its limitations though:

(a) The results can be very sensitive to the performance ratings and thus to differences in judgement-based scores or errors in the data.
(b) The resulting shortlist will include the best option but a shortlist of five, say, will not necessarily consist of the best five options. Like an unseeded knock-out competition, a good candidate may be eliminated early in the process by a slightly better one.
(c) Generally there will be very few dominated options unless there are large numbers of tied scores. This may not occur unless the scoring systems are fairly insensitive.

Nonetheless, it can be a very useful first step, and it may be possible to eliminate more options by examining specific pairs and debating the necessary trade-offs. If Option A has major advantages in terms of criteria 1, 2 and 3, and Option B has only minor advantages in terms of criterion 4, criterion 4 would have to be very important for B to be worth considering further. This is an example of what Hammond and colleagues (1999) call 'practical dominance' of B by A.

## Weighting methods

Satisficing would have eliminated 11 of the options in Table 4.2 and left 9. You could have taken this as a starting point for using weighting or sequential elimination but your decision making group have decided that a 'poor' on one criterion should not be enough to reject an option if it does well in other respects.

Now you are going to try using weights on the full set of 20. Remember that the first stage in a weightings-based analysis is conversion of the performance ratings into *interval* scores. Some of the work has been done for you in the preparation of Table 4.3. This has been derived from Table 4.2 by coding good = 2, fair = 1 and poor = 0. Also running costs in Table 4.2 have been subtracted from a notional £3m and capital costs subtracted from £6m so that the cost figures in Table 4.3 can be seen as savings against notional sums.

### Converting performance ratings to preference scores

As you have already learned, the set of performance ratings for each criterion (e.g. all the ratings for staff acceptability) need to be converted to 'equal interval' preference scores. Now you will learn how to do this.

The first step is to anchor the scale by choosing reference points. In Table 4.3, the worst option is scored at the bottom of the range (at zero, say) and the best option is scored at the top. This is called local scaling. For the first three criteria in the table, this is easy. The options rated poor and scoring zero are at the bottom of the scale and those rated good and scoring 2 are at the top.

Once you have anchored your scale, the position of each intermediate option has to be worked out. For the first three criteria this task is relatively easy to describe, if

**Table 4.3** Scores derived from ratings as a basis for weighted analysis

| Site | Staff acceptability | Accessibility for patients | Quality of environment | Running costs £ | Capital cost £ |
|------|------|------|------|------|------|
| 1 | 2 | 1 | 0 | 1300 | 3000 |
| 2 | 1 | 1 | 2 | 700 | 2200 |
| 3 | 0 | 1 | 1 | 900 | 1800 |
| 4 | 1 | 2 | 1 | 1800 | 800 |
| 5 | 0 | 1 | 1 | 900 | 4600 |
| 6 | 2 | 2 | 2 | 1200 | 2200 |
| 7 | 2 | 0 | 2 | 2200 | 1800 |
| 8 | 1 | 0 | 1 | 2300 | 1000 |
| 9 | 1 | 1 | 1 | 1200 | 2000 |
| 10 | 2 | 2 | 2 | 2000 | 1200 |
| 11 | 2 | 1 | 2 | 900 | 2300 |
| 12 | 1 | 2 | 1 | 1900 | 600 |
| 13 | 0 | 1 | 1 | 1300 | 4000 |
| 14 | 1 | 2 | 2 | 500 | 2000 |
| 15 | 0 | 2 | 1 | 1200 | 3600 |
| 16 | 0 | 1 | 0 | 900 | 4000 |
| 17 | 0 | 2 | 2 | 1400 | 4600 |
| 18 | 1 | 0 | 2 | 2400 | 4100 |
| 19 | 1 | 0 | 1 | 2300 | 2600 |
| 20 | 2 | 1 | 1 | 1800 | 1000 |

not to accomplish. It comes down to the question of whether the options rated fair and scoring one are actually at the middle of the scale in preference terms. Or are they above or below the middle? And if so, by how much?

The cost criteria are more difficult, partly because they are more evenly spread over a range but mainly because the range of ratings is much wider. Unless you take this into account, costs will completely overwhelm everything else in a weighted analysis because, for example, capital costs differ between the best and the worst options from 4600 to 600 = 4000, compared to 2 – 0 = 2 for the others.

The most common approach is to rescale the ratings so that the scores for the best option on each criterion are all the same and the scores for the worst options over all the same. In Table 4.4, all the scores for all the criteria have been rescaled so that they fall into the range 0 to 2, but a range of 0 to 100 is more common.

This leaves you with the question of whether the cost scores actually measure preferences. Option 19 scores 1 on capital costs because its rating of 2600 is midway between the best (Option 5) and worst (Option 12). But is Option 5 preferred to Option 19 by the same amount as Option 19 is preferred to Option 12? If so you can use the rescaled ratings in Table 4.4 as preference scores in a weighted analysis. If not, consensus judgements will be needed to make adjustments.

A variation on this approach involves fixing the bottom of the scale as the worst *possible* option ever likely to be considered and the top as the best possible. This is called global (as opposed to local) scaling. Its advantage is that it allows options that are better or worse in some respects than any of the current set to be added to the analysis later. Its disadvantage is that to fix the reference points, you have the

**Table 4.4** Rescaled ratings: a step towards preference scores as a basis for weighted analysis

| Site | Staff acceptability | Accessibility for patients | Quality of environment | Running costs £ | Capital cost £ |
|---|---|---|---|---|---|
| 1 | 2 | 1 | 0 | 0.8 | 1.2 |
| 2 | 1 | 1 | 2 | 0.2 | 0.8 |
| 3 | 0 | 1 | 1 | 0.4 | 0.6 |
| 4 | 1 | 2 | 1 | 1.4 | 0.1 |
| 5 | 0 | 1 | 1 | 0.4 | 2 |
| 6 | 2 | 2 | 2 | 0.7 | 0.8 |
| 7 | 2 | 0 | 2 | 1.8 | 0.6 |
| 8 | 1 | 0 | 1 | 1.9 | 0.2 |
| 9 | 1 | 1 | 1 | 0.7 | 0.7 |
| 10 | 2 | 2 | 2 | 1.6 | 0.3 |
| 11 | 2 | 1 | 2 | 0.4 | 0.9 |
| 12 | 1 | 2 | 1 | 1.5 | 0 |
| 13 | 0 | 1 | 1 | 0.8 | 1.7 |
| 14 | 1 | 2 | 2 | 0 | 0.7 |
| 15 | 0 | 2 | 1 | 0.7 | 1.5 |
| 16 | 0 | 1 | 0 | 0.4 | 1.7 |
| 17 | 0 | 2 | 2 | 0.9 | 2 |
| 18 | 1 | 0 | 2 | 2 | 1.8 |
| 19 | 1 | 0 | 1 | 1.9 | 1.0 |
| 20 | 2 | 1 | 1 | 1.4 | 0.2 |

additional problem of deciding what the hypothetical worst and best possible options might be like. They may be hard to imagine and even harder to agree upon.

## An approach to deriving 'importance' weights for criteria: 'swing weighting'

Now you are ready to think about ways of deriving 'importance' weights for your criteria. First, determine the criterion with the biggest difference in preference between the top and bottom of the scale. This criterion is assigned a weight of 100 and becomes the standard. Suppose the biggest difference in preference is between the best and worst options in terms of running cost.

The swings in preference between the ends of the scales for the other criteria are then judged in comparison with this standard and assigned values between 0 and 100. For staff acceptability there may be relatively little difference between the best and worst options, so this criterion might be assigned a weight of 35. The best and worst options for patient acceptability might be a bit further apart, suggesting a weight of 45. And so on. This might be done as a nominal group exercise, with each participant making their own private ratings and then taking part in a discussion about areas of disagreement. If reasonable agreement is beyond reach, different sets of weights may be tried in a sensitivity analysis.

**Activity 4.5**

Once you have a set of weights, they are usually rescaled to add up to one. Suppose that after rescaling your importance weights are as follows:

| | |
|---|---|
| Acceptability to staff | 0.15 |
| Accessibility for patients | 0.25 |
| Environmental quality | 0.05 |
| Running costs | 0.45 |
| Capital costs | 0.10 |

Which options come out best? And which come out worst?

**Feedback**

The results of the weighting process can be seen in Table 4.5. Option 10 is fairly comfortably the best. Its capital cost is high but this is given relatively little weight. Options 12 and 4 are second and third, with not much between them; again, both have high capital costs. Option 3 is the worst.

**Table 4.5** Sites for the health centre with weighted sums of scores and ranks

| Site weight | Staff acceptability 0.150 | Accessibility for patients 0.250 | Quality of environment 0.050 | Running costs 0.450 | Capital cost 0.100 | Weighted sum | Rank of weighted sum |
|---|---|---|---|---|---|---|---|
| 1 | 2 | 1 | 0 | 0.8 | 1.2 | 1.05 | 11 |
| 2 | 1 | 1 | 2 | 0.2 | 0.8 | 0.67 | 18 |
| 3 | 0 | 1 | 1 | 0.4 | 0.6 | 0.55 | 20 |
| 4 | 1 | 2 | 1 | 1.4 | 0.1 | 1.33 | 3 |
| 5 | 0 | 1 | 1 | 0.4 | 2.0 | 0.69 | 17 |
| 6 | 2 | 2 | 2 | 0.7 | 0.8 | 1.31 | 5 |
| 7 | 2 | 0 | 2 | 1.8 | 0.6 | 1.27 | 6 |
| 8 | 1 | 0 | 1 | 1.9 | 0.2 | 1.07 | 10 |
| 9 | 1 | 1 | 1 | 0.7 | 0.7 | 0.85 | 14 |
| 10 | 2 | 2 | 2 | 1.6 | 0.3 | 1.64 | 1 |
| 11 | 2 | 1 | 2 | 0.4 | 0.9 | 0.92 | 13 |
| 12 | 1 | 2 | 1 | 1.5 | 0.0 | 1.36 | 2 |
| 13 | 0 | 1 | 1 | 0.8 | 1.7 | 0.85 | 15 |
| 14 | 1 | 2 | 2 | 0.0 | 0.7 | 0.82 | 16 |
| 15 | 0 | 2 | 1 | 0.7 | 1.5 | 1.03 | 12 |
| 16 | 0 | 1 | 0 | 0.4 | 1.7 | 0.61 | 19 |
| 17 | 0 | 2 | 2 | 0.9 | 2.0 | 1.23 | 8 |
| 18 | 1 | 0 | 2 | 2.0 | 1.8 | 1.33 | 4 |
| 19 | 1 | 0 | 1 | 1.9 | 1.0 | 1.15 | 9 |
| 20 | 2 | 1 | 1 | 1.4 | 0.2 | 1.24 | 7 |

## Sequential elimination

You have seen that weighting methods involve a lot of judgements. Many people feel uncomfortable making judgements of these kinds. They may feel that the judgements themselves are arbitrary, but there may be other reasons. They may feel uncertain about a process that they do not really understand or trust. For example, they may feel that some of their colleagues may have been cheating by assigning high importance weights to criteria that support an option that they favour for some quite different reason!

 **Activity 4.6**

Return to Table 4.3 and try sequential or pairwise elimination. Identify dominated options and eliminate them from the table.

 **Feedback**

The following options are dominated:

- Sites 3 and 16 are dominated by, for example, Site 5. (Site 3 is in fact dominated by seven other sites.)
- Sites 2, 9 and 14 are dominated by Site 6.
- Sites 4, 12, and 20 are dominated by Site 10.
- Sites 5, 13 and 15 are dominated by Site 17.
- Sites 8 and 19 are dominated by Site 18.

Eliminating the dominated decision options reduces the number of sites for the location of the health centre from 20 to 7. The remaining sites are shown in Table 4.6.

**Table 4.6** Health centre sites remaining after eliminating dominated options

| Site | Staff acceptability | Accessibility for patients | Quality of environment | Running costs | Capital cost |
|------|------|------|------|------|------|
| 1  | 2 | 1 | 0 | 1300 | 3000 |
| 6  | 2 | 2 | 2 | 1200 | 2200 |
| 7  | 2 | 0 | 2 | 2200 | 1800 |
| 10 | 2 | 2 | 2 | 2000 | 1200 |
| 11 | 2 | 1 | 2 | 900  | 2300 |
| 17 | 0 | 2 | 2 | 1400 | 4600 |
| 18 | 1 | 0 | 2 | 2400 | 4100 |

## Ways of going further

Sequential elimination has been helpful in the case of Activity 4.6, largely because three of the five criteria were rated very crudely, so there was a high proportion of ties. But there are seven options left, and still some way to go. In some decision problems there may be no dominated options.

There are a number of possible ways forward. One intuitive approach is to allow options to be eliminated if they are almost dominated. Compare Options 6 and 11, for example. They rate the same on staff acceptability and environment. Option 6 is better on patient accessibility (2 vs 1) and running costs (1200 vs 900). Option 11 is slightly better on running costs (2300 vs 2200). On this basis the decision makers might informally agree to eliminate Option 11.

You will learn about two more formal approaches, one based exclusively on pairwise comparisons, and one using a combination of pairwise comparisons and importance weights for the criteria. Finally, you will learn about a way of deriving importance weights using paired comparisons.

## Even swaps

Hammond and colleagues (1999) describe an approach to making trade-offs between scores on different criteria based on specific pairwise comparisons called 'even swaps'. This is a more formal approach to the kind of judgement just made when eliminating Option 11. Making an even swap involves increasing the value of an option in terms of one criterion while decreasing its value *by an equivalent amount* in terms of another.

In Table 4.6, consider Option 1. If its score on 'quality of environment' were increased from 0 to 2, there would be no difference between any of the options according to this criterion. This would mean that you could simplify the problem by dropping the environmental criterion, and this may lead to more dominated options. Suppose that the decision makers were offered a version of Option 1 (called Option 1a, say) with its environmental rating increased from 0 to 2 but capital cost rating reduced to compensate. Suppose that a capital rating for Option 1a of only 1100 instead of 3000 would make Options 1 and 1a equally preferred, or an 'even swap'. Would Option 1a survive in Table 4.6? With this capital rating, it would be dominated by Option 10. But the decision makers regard Options 1 and 1a as equivalent in terms of preference, so to be consistent they should prefer Option 10 to Option 1 as well. On this basis there is a case for eliminating Option 1.

Next the decision makers might devise Option 17a, which is in many respects the same as Option 17 but has a staff acceptability rating of 2 instead of 0. For Options 17 and 17a to be an even swap, the decision makers consider that 17a's capital cost rating would have to come down to about 1000. In that case it, too, would be dominated by Option 10. If, on the other hand, 17a's capital cost rating were still up at around 2500, it would dominate Options 6 and 11. This would leave just four Options (7, 10, 17 and 18) to choose from.

It might be possible to carry on working through the performance matrix in a systematic way until only one option remains. This may involve some difficult choices but the process is transparent, manageable and grounded in direct comparisons between options, even if some of them are artificial.

## Outranking

Roy (1996) has suggested another approach to pairwise comparison based on what he calls 'outranking relations'. He redefines dominance in a less demanding way than is conventional: Option A is said to outrank Option B if A is at least as good as B on enough criteria of *enough importance* and is not seriously worse than B in any respect. This method is more demanding than even swaps in that it requires 'importance' weights for the different criteria but generally requires fewer judgement-based comparisons.

The first test – enough criteria of enough importance – is assessed by a *concordance index*, which is simply the sum of the weights for the criteria on which A scores at least as highly as B.

The second test, which acts as a kind of veto on the concordance index in cases where an option performs particularly badly, even if only in one respect, is assessment by a *discordance index*. Calculation of this is more complex but if you are interested in finding out more, the formulae and some results can be seen in the file on your CD called Ch4MulCrit! on the spreadsheet called 'Outranking'.

It is up to the decision makers to adjust the power of the analysis to discriminate, by choosing threshold values for the two indices. To see how this works, look at the spreadsheet. Assume the same set of criterion importance weights as in Activity 4.5 (Table 4.5) and the shortlist of options in Table 4.6. Choose the threshold values 0.85 and 0.80 for the concordance and discordance indexes, in cells S6 and S18 respectively. It can be seen from the range AB30:AB36 in the spreadsheet that Option 1 is again eliminated following comparison with Option 10. However, Option 17 is also eliminated, because it ranks so poorly on staff acceptability. Lowering the discordance threshold to 0.70 leads to Option 11 being eliminated by Option 10, and with concordance threshold at 0.70, Option 7 becomes dominated by Option 18. At this stage only Options 6, 10 and 18 remain.

## The Analytical Hierarchy Process: importance weights based on pairwise preferences

The relative transparency of pairwise comparisons of options suggests that decision makers may find it easier to derive importance weights for criteria from pairwise comparisons of criteria than direct judgements. One method of doing this is part of a broader approach to multiple criteria decision making called the Analytical Hierarchy Process (AHP) (Saaty 1980). Similar methods may be used for determining option scores.

This involves an agreed scale for the comparison of pairs of criteria (criterion A and criterion B, say). Commonly a 9-point scale is used. The odd-numbered scale points are labelled, with the values of the interspersed even-numbered points left implicit:

1 = A and B equally preferred (i.e. to be given equal weight).
3 = A moderately preferred to B.
5 = A strongly preferred.
7 = A very strongly preferred.
9 = A extremely strongly preferred.

Part of this method is that if the score of A relative to B is 3, then the score of B relative to A is defined as 1/3.

On this basis the group might construct a pairwise comparison matrix that looks like Table 4.7. This shows that, for example, acceptability to staff is considered about as important as accessibility to patients, but 'moderately' more important than environmental quality.

**Table 4.7** A pairwise comparison matrix

| Criterion | Acceptable | Access | Environment | Running | Capital |
|---|---|---|---|---|---|
| Acceptability to staff | 1 | 1 | 3 | 1/3 | 1 |
| Accessibility for patients | 1 | 1 | 5 | 1/2 | 1 |
| Environmental quality | 1/3 | 1/5 | 1 | 1/7 | 1/2 |
| Running cost | 3 | 2 | 7 | 1 | 5 |
| Capital cost | 1 | 1 | 2 | 1/5 | 1 |

Saaty's method of constructing weights from this set of preferences involves matrix computations that are beyond the scope of this book. A simple approximate method is used in the spreadsheet called AHP in Ch4MulCrit! and you can examine the formulae involved there.

The weights that come out of this add up to 1.0 and are as follows:

| | |
|---|---|
| Acceptability to staff | 0.16 |
| Accessibility for patients | 0.20 |
| Environmental quality | 0.05 |
| Running cost | 0.46 |
| Capital cost | 0.13 |

The AHP has been criticized because it allows participants to choose inconsistent sets of weights. Suppose that the preference score for A over B was 3, and for B over C it was 4. The implication is that the preference score for A over C should be 12 but this is off the scale, which has a maximum of 10! Also consistency would require that if equal weight is given to Acceptability and Accessibility, say, then the weightings of these two criteria relative to others should be the same. In Table 4.7, Acceptability is moderately preferred to Environmental quality, but Accessibility is strongly preferred to it, so there is an inconsistency there. In severe cases, adding a new option to the analysis can change the relative ranking of some of the original options, which makes no sense.

To address this criticism, AHP involves use of a 'consistency index'. How this is calculated is also shown on spreadsheet 'AHP' in Ch4MulCrit!. In this case the index value is 0.029. The index for a randomly generated preference matrix with five criteria would be 1.12, and 0.029/1.12 is considered well within the satisfactory level of 0.10. Above this kind of level, the amount of inconsistency in the table would be considered problematic, and any results suspect.

This approach does have a number of advantages over less formal methods. It is reasonably transparent; it requires relatively limited judgements by the participants; it generally gives plausible results; and it includes a method of assessing consistency.

On the other hand, it depends on the decision making group agreeing on a set of preference ratings. While this is asking less than agreement about weights, even this may not be possible. Special-purpose software is available which simplifies the task of carrying out sensitivity analyses on the preference matrix, which may or may not help.

## Pros and cons of multiple criteria decision methods in general

In a very useful manual on the subject produced for a British government department (DTLR 2000), the advantages of multiple criteria decision analysis over informal unsupported judgement are given as follows:

- It is open and explicit.
- The choice of objectives and criteria that any decision making group may make are open to analysis and to change if they are felt to be inappropriate.
- Scores and weights, when used, are also explicit and are developed according to established techniques. They can also be cross-referenced to other sources of information on relative values and amended if necessary.
- Performance measurement can be sub-contracted to experts, so need not necessarily be left in the hands of the decision making body itself.
- It can provide an important means of communication, within the decision making body and sometimes, later, between that body and the wider community.
- Scores and weights are used which provide an audit trail.

On the one hand, you have seen some of the difficulties with weighting methods. Essentially these are arriving at an agreed and properly scaled set of preference scores and arriving at an agreed set of criterion weights. Sequential elimination or pairwise comparison is generally easier to do and often good progress can be made without have to make trade-offs, towards shortlisting at least. On the other hand, the latter stages of the elimination process may become increasingly controversial and sensitivity analysis is more difficult than weighting methods.

## Summary

In this chapter you have learned how to structure a decision making problem with multiple criteria. You have been introduced to a number of concepts and approaches, including the performance matrix; ratings, preference scores and importance weights for criteria; satisficing, sequential elimination and weighting; dominance and outranking.

## References

Cushman M and Rosenhead J (2004) Planning in the face of politics: reshaping children's health services in Inner London, in Brandeau M, Sainfort F and Pierskalla W (eds) *Operations Research and Health Care: A Handbook of Methods and Applications*. Boston: Kluwer Academic Publishers.

DTLR (2000) Multi-criteria analysis manual section 4.3.1 www.odpm.gov.uk/stellent/groups/
odpm_about/documents/source/odpm_about_source_608524.doc

Friend J and Hickling A (eds) (2004) *The Strategic Choice Approach* (3rd edn). Oxford: Architectural Press.

Hammond JS, Keeney RL and Raiffa H (1999) *Smart Choices: A Practical Guide to Making Better
Decisions*. Boston, MA: Harvard Business School Press.

Roy B (1996) *Multi-criteria Methodology for Decision Aiding*. Dordrecht: Kluwer.

Saaty T (1980) *The Analytical Hierarchy Process*. New York: John Wiley.

# Uncertainty

## Overview

You have already come across uncertainty about values, and you learned about methods for addressing these in Chapters 3 and 4. In this chapter you will learn about three methods for dealing with uncertainty about outcomes. One is *game theory*, which offers a number of strategies that reflect different attitudes to uncertainty. The second is *robustness analysis*, which is based on the idea that in an uncertain world it is better, if possible, to make a sequence of decisions that preserve flexibility by keeping as many good options open as you can, than to make one inflexible decision that may be overtaken by events. The third is AIDA (analysis of interconnected decision areas).

## Learning objectives

**By the end of this chapter, you will be better able to:**

- **distinguish between different aspects of uncertainty in decision making, including uncertainty about the working environment, about values and about related agendas**
- **describe strategies from game theory for dealing with uncertainty arising from lack of knowledge or factors beyond the decision maker's control**
- **describe the principles of robustness analysis when there is uncertainty about the future and the decision problem can be broken down into a sequence so as to keep options open**
- **describe the principles of analysing interconnected decision areas when there is uncertainty about related agendas**

## Key terms

**Decision area** Any area of choice within which decision makers can conceive of an alternative course of action that might be adopted, now or at some future time.

**Payoff** In a single-criterion decision problem, the outcome or value of a given decision option for a given state of nature.

**Regret** For a given state of nature, the loss of payoff associated with a given decision option when compared with what would have been the payoff from the best decision option.

**States of nature** Possible combinations of events and circumstances that are beyond the control of the decision makers (i.e. determined by exogenous variables).

## Introduction: What is uncertainty?

In the last chapter, uncertainty was identified as one of the factors that made decision making difficult. Daellenbach (2002) characterizes it as follows:

 **Uncertainty**

Uncertainty refers to incomplete knowledge about something – an event, a phenomenon, a process, a future outcome, or something in the past that has not been revealed fully. The uncertainty could be about the attribute(s) of something, e.g. its gender, or its numeric value, or its timing. The degree of uncertainty may vary from knowing almost nothing, e.g. we only have a partial list of potential outcomes, to knowing almost everything, e.g. we may know that its numeric value lies inside a narrow band.

Uncertainty is an everyday occurrence and we have many words related to the concept: chance, likelihood, probability, risk, hazard, random, stochastic, odds, to name just a few. What are the causes of uncertainty?

- *Ignorance:* The thing is not understood in sufficient detail. If we completely understood the processes that cause earthquakes, we could predict the timing and severity of the next earthquake occurring in San Francisco.
- *Incomplete information:* It is technically possible to get complete information, but for various reasons, such as limited funds or time, we only collect information about a sample of the thing. For instance, TV ratings for various programmes are based on a small fraction of all viewers. Hence they are inaccurate. It is again ignorance, but by design.
- *Inability to predict the moves of other parties involved:* The final outcome of a process may be the joint result of actions taken by competing parties – economic competitors, opposing teams. Their actions or moves may be taken independently of each other or in response to or anticipation of the competitors' moves.
- *Measurement errors:* They may be due to mistakes made by observers or inaccuracies in the measuring instruments.

In the context of decision making, the most obvious problem is uncertainty about *outcomes*. You are uncertain about what might happen if you decide to do X rather than Y, because there are factors that you do not know enough about or are beyond your control. Daellenbach points out the distinction commonly made in the literature between decision making in a situation involving *complete* uncertainty and in a situation involving *risk:*

- *uncertainty* implies that you know what possible outcomes might be but have no information about the likelihood of each;
- *risk* implies knowledge about the probability of each outcome.

In this chapter you will learn about approaches to analysing decisions that assume no knowledge of the probabilities of the different possible outcomes. In some circumstances this is a strength, but if there is a sufficient basis for estimates of risk, it is a weakness. In the next chapter you will learn about methods that incorporate estimates of the probabilities of the different outcomes.

## Uncertainty, one decision point and one criterion: game theory

In Chapter 4 you were a member of a team responsible for the provision of health care for the population of a given area. You had to decide where to build a new health centre, taking into account five criteria. Now imagine that one way or another you have reduced the list of options to three sites in different towns labelled X, Y and Z. The three sites are known to be similar in terms of all five criteria except their accessibility to populations of patients. Thus you now have what is effectively a one-criterion problem, which would be relatively simple if you knew how accessible each option would be.

However, in some circumstances it is not clear which site will turn out best in terms of improving accessibility. Suppose there has been a rumour that a factory in town Z, which is the major local employer, might be closed down and manufacturing concentrated in the company's factory in town Y. It has been impossible to get any clarification of this from either local management or head office, which is in another country. Also town Z is quite near the border of the area for which you are responsible. Just over the border is another town and there is some uncertainty over whether your counterparts in the neighbouring health care organization intend to build a new health centre there. If they did, it would draw off some of Town Z's (and also some of Town X's) health centre catchment population. You have suggested a joint planning exercise but your counterparts are in the middle of organizational restructuring and say that they have not got time to discuss this, and cannot make any long-term commitments.

### States of nature

The first step is to identify the set of possible *states of nature* or 'environmental' scenarios. These are the possible sets of circumstances that are beyond your control but could affect how well your decision turns out. This set should be mutually exclusive (i.e. one state of nature cannot exist at the same time as another) and exhaustive (i.e. all possible states of nature are covered).

In this case, there are two propositions that you are uncertain about:

A  The factory in Town Z will move to Town Y.
B  A new health centre will be built over the border from Towns Z and X.

This gives you four environmental scenarios: E1 (neither A nor B); E2 (A but not B); E3 (B but not A); and E4 (both A and B).

The decision problem thus involves three options and four scenarios. Each scenario could occur with each option, so there are 12 possible *outcomes* to consider. Assume that you can summarize your views about the relative desirability of each outcome in terms of a single *payoff* or desirability score. Thus instead of the single preference scores for each option that you had in the performance matrices in Chapter 4 where there was no allowance for uncertainty, you now have four scenario-dependent payoffs. These are set out in a *payoff matrix* in Table 5.1. Nothing is known about which of the four environmental scenarios is most likely. Which site should be chosen?

**Table 5.1** The payoff matrix for a decision making problem under uncertainty

| Choices | Possible environmental scenarios | | | |
|---|---|---|---|---|
|  | E1 | E2 | E3 | E4 |
| X | 7 | 3 | 4 | 0 |
| Y | 2 | 2 | 5 | 5 |
| Z | 10 | 5 | 3 | −2 |

### Strategies for making a choice

*Game theory* suggests a number of possible strategies for making a choice. Here you learn about three of them.

1 *Maximax*: For Site X, the maximum payoff is 7, occurring under scenario E1. For Site Y the maximum is 5 (E3 and E4), and for Site Z the maximum is 10 (E1). The maximax strategy is to pick the option that gives the *max*imum of the *max*imum payoffs; in this case you would choose Site Z because it gives 10. This is a strategy for the optimistic or risk-prone decision maker; as far as we know, E4 is just as likely as E1, and could be much more so, in which case choosing Site Z may well turn out to have been disastrous.

2 *Maximin*: For Site X, the worst that can happen is E4; this gives the minimum payoff of 0. The minimum payoffs for Sites Y and Z are 2 (under E1 and E2) and −2 (under E4) respectively. So the best (or *max*imum) of the *min*imum payoffs is 2, which arises from choosing Site Y. This *maximin* strategy is for the pessimistic or risk-averse decision maker. It assumes that whatever site you choose, the worst will happen.

3 *Minimax regret*. For this strategy you need to derive a *regret* matrix from your payoff matrix. How is this done? Suppose that E1 turns out to be the scenario that actually occurs. The best decision would have been to go for Site Z (payoff = 10). Having chosen Site X though, the payoff is only 7, so that the amount of regret felt by anyone who chose Site X and then *had to put up with E1* would be 10 − 7, or 3. This is shown in Table 5.2. Similarly, the amount of regret involved in having chosen Site Y and then living through E2 is 5 − 2 = 3. Now, check for yourself that the greatest (maximum) regret that could result from having chosen Site X is 5 (under E4); the maximum regret for Site Y is 8 (under E1) and for Site Z it is 7 (under E4). Under the *minimax regret* strategy you choose Site X, because you want to *min*imize the *max*imum amount of regret that could occur, given your choice. This is a strategy for decision makers who want to minimize disappointment or criticism of their decision after the event.

**Table 5.2** The regret matrix derived from the payoff matrix in Table 5.1

| Choice | Possible environmental scenarios | | | |
|---|---|---|---|---|
|  | E1 | E2 | E3 | E4 |
| X | 3 | 2 | 1 | 5 |
| Y | 8 | 3 | 0 | 0 |
| Z | 0 | 0 | 2 | 7 |

Now try this out yourself using a different example. Return to your first decision making problem in Chapter 4, about extending an operating theatre block. Suppose that it is known that a neighbouring hospital is also considering extending its theatre block. If they do, the demand for surgery at your hospital will be reduced. Also, a recent policy document recommends increasing the volume of day surgery but it is not clear how surgeons will receive this report. If they accept all its recommendations, then there would be a significant increase in the percentage of surgery done on a day care basis and a reduction in demand for inpatient surgery. There is already a theatre for day surgery which is working below its capacity.

Estimates of the demand for in-patient surgery at your hospital (in thousands of operations) under different states of nature are: for day surgery report accepted, = 11 if neighbouring hospital expands = 11 and 15 if it does not expand; for day surgery report not accepted the corresponding figures are 13 and 16 respectively.

Remember that currently the hospital has the capacity to perform 12,000 operations per year and that your management are considering building up to another two theatres, each with a capacity of 2000 operations per year.

 **Activity 5.1**

Identify the *mutually exclusive* states of nature involved. Then using the above information calculate the differences between inpatient theatre capacity and estimated demand when 0, 1, or 2 operating theatres are built, for each state of nature.

 **Feedback**

There are two exogenous variables. Each will take one of two possible values:

• neighbour expands? yes/no
• report is accepted? yes/no

The decision options (determining capacity) and the states of nature (determining demand) are shown in Table 5.3.

**Table 5.3** New operating theatres – capacity and demand

| Number of theatres built | Capacity (000s) | Estimated demand (000s) | | | |
|---|---|---|---|---|---|
| | | Neighbour does not expand, report not accepted | Neighbour expands, report not accepted | Neighbour does not expand, report accepted | Neighbour expands, report accepted |
| 0 | 12 | 16 | 13 | 15 | 11 |
| 1 | 14 | 16 | 13 | 15 | 11 |
| 2 | 16 | 16 | 13 | 15 | 11 |

The difference between capacity and demand is shown in Table 5.4; negative numbers indicate capacity below demand, positive numbers indicate capacity above demand.

**Table 5.4** New operating theatres – difference between capacity and demand

| | Difference between capacity and demand (000s) | | | |
|---|---|---|---|---|
| Number of theatres built | Neighbour does not expand, report not accepted | Neighbour expands, report not accepted | Neighbour does not expand, report accepted | Neighbour expands, report accepted |
| 0 | –4 | –1 | –3 | 1 |
| 1 | –2 | 1 | –1 | 3 |
| 2 | 0 | 3 | 1 | 5 |

 **Activity 5.2**

Now construct a payoff matrix. To do this, assume that the payoff for each combination of options and states of nature is proportional to the difference between capacity and demand, which you calculated in Activity 5.1. Over-capacity of 1000 operations is regarded as *just as undesirable* as under-capacity of 1000 operations, so that the greater the *absolute value* of the difference between capacity and demand, the worse the payoff.

**Feedback**

In this case a difference of 1000 between capacity and demand can be scored as a utility of minus 1. Table 5.5 gives the results.

**Table 5.5** New operating theatres – payoff matrix

| | E1 | E2 | E3 | E4 |
|---|---|---|---|---|
| build 0 | –4 | –1 | –3 | –1 |
| build 1 | –2 | –1 | –1 | –3 |
| build 2 | 0 | –3 | –1 | –5 |

For the purposes of this exercise a rather crude approach to measuring utility has been used. Another approach would have been to construct the payoff matrix by seeking the consensus among interested parties on the relative desirability of each option/scenario combination.

This approach is awkward as well as crude because the *greater* the absolute value of the difference between capacity and demand, the worse the outcome, whereas our decision strategies are based on higher payoffs being better. One way of dealing with this is to make all utilities negative. This has been done in Table 5.5. (The other way is to substitute minimization for maximization, and vice versa, in the strategies you use, so that maximax becomes minimin etc., but this can be even more confusing!)

**Activity 5.3**

What are the maximax, maximin, and minimax regret solutions to this problem? (If you use Excel to perform the calculations, you can use the built-in functions MAX() and MIN() to identify the best and worst payoffs respectively. These functions accept a range of cells as an argument. Thus MAX(Z4:Z10) gives you the maximum of the values in the cells Z4 to Z10.)

 **Feedback**

The maximax strategy suggests building two theatres, because 0 is the maximum of the values (−1,−1,0), which are the least bad payoffs for the three options respectively. The maximin strategy suggests building one theatre because −3 is the least bad of the values (−4,−3,−5) which are the worst payoffs for each option under any scenario.

The regrets matrix is shown in Table 5.6. The maximum (worst) regrets for each option under any scenario are 4, 2 and 4 for Options 1, 2 and 3 respectively. Thus the minimax regret strategy also suggests Option 2, building one theatre, because 2 is the minimum of the maximum regrets.

**Table 5.6** New operating theatres: the regrets matrix

|         | E1 | E2 | E3 | E4 |
|---------|----|----|----|----|
| build 0 | 4  | 0  | 2  | 0  |
| build 1 | 2  | 0  | 0  | 2  |
| build 2 | 0  | 2  | 0  | 4  |

## Some shortcomings of game theory approach

This approach, based on *game theory* has two main shortcomings:

1  Real decision problems usually involve many criteria, and this approach is based on a single payoff score. One way round this is to use the techniques you learned about in Chapter 4 for converting a set of performance ratings into a single score using preference scores and criterion weights, or maybe using direct judgements. The effect of bringing in uncertainty is that the performance ratings depend on the future state of nature as well as the option chosen.

2  One of its defining features is that it does not incorporate any information you may have about the likelihood of the different scenarios or states of nature. In general, only the extreme values of payoff in the matrix (the minimum and maximum in any row or column) can influence the decision. Thus the approach often does not exploit all the information available.

In Chapter 6 you will consider another single-criterion approach. This *requires* estimates of the likelihood of the various possible states of nature and uses all the information in the payoff matrix.

## Sequential decisions and robustness analysis

In the last problem, one of the sources of uncertainty was how the surgeons would respond to the report on day surgery. Instead of making a final decision at this stage, one way forward might be to build just one new operating theatre and then wait and see what happened to demand. If one theatre was not enough, you could then build a second. This is not necessarily a good idea because it might be much more expensive to build in two phases, but it would be worth exploring. As Rosenhead (2001) points out:

> The future is necessarily a combination of the known and the unknowable. The proportion of the latter tends to rise as the time-scale extends, graphically represented by the 'trumpet of uncertainty' opening out into a wide bell . . .
>
> Longer term or strategic planning cannot be firmly based on an attempt to predict what *will* happen, rendered infeasible as it is by the purposeful interactions of other human and social actors. A more limited task, of identifying a range of versions of what *might* happen, would be a modest and supportable basis for planning analysis.

Where you can, it is sensible to avoid making a big decision that determines the configuration of services for some time into the future but rather make a sequence of smaller decisions. Decisions early in the sequence that maintain flexibility and keep options open allow later decisions to take events into account as they unfold. Rosenhead proposes an approach which he calls robustness analysis, in which early decisions are good if they keep good options open.

 ### Robustness analysis

There is more than one possible strategy when confronted by high levels of uncertainty . . . One might be to attempt to control the environment from which the uncertainty emanates. Another is to tighten up internal organization for quicker response when unpredicted change occurs. However, when none of these strategies is available, or in addition to them, ensuring flexibility may avoid untoward consequences. Indeed it may make it possible to take advantage of unexpected opportunities: the eventual manifestations of uncertainty are not always malign.

Once the unexpected has occurred, it can be straightforward to see how policy or position should be modified. Such modification may, however, be impossible without damaging costs or sacrifice of other desiderata. How serious the consequences of change to meet the new conditions are will depend on how easily the previous posture can accommodate the necessary transformations.

Such flexibility may turn out to be available when demands on it are made. However, it is more prudent to attempt to *engineer* a high level of flexibility rather than rely on lucky accidents. Liquidity (in financial management), versatility (of military forces), resilience (of ecological systems) and hedging (in the planning of investments) are all analytic tools developed in different planning environments to achieve this flexible capability.

'Robustness', and the analysis based on it, embodies a particular perspective on flexibility. It is concerned with situations where an individual, group or organization needs to make commitments now under conditions of uncertainty, and where these decisions will be followed at intervals by other commitments. With a robustness perspective the focus will be on the alternative immediate commitments which could be made, which will be compared in terms of the range of possible future commitments with which they appear to be compatible.

The distinctive features of this perspective are brought out in Figure 5.1. This represents schematically the classical 'planning-as-decision making' approach: an optimal system for an assumed future state of the environment is derived, and the plan consists of the necessary decisions required to transform the current system into that target configuration.

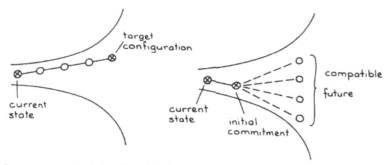

Robustness analysis is a bifocal instrument.

(a) classical planning methodology     (b) robustness methodology

**Figure 5.1** Planning and the trumpet of uncertainty

Source: Rosenhead (2001).

The robustness methodology in Figure 5.1(b) by contrast declines to identify a future decision path or target. The only firm commitments called for are those in the initial decision package – possible future commitments are of interest principally for the range of capability to respond to unexpected developments in the environment which they represent. (The term 'decision package' is used to indicate that initial commitments may come in integrated bundles.)

Graphical illustrations suggest but do not define a method. A more formal measure of the options left open is required, if initial commitments are to be compared to see which is the more robust. We define the *robustness* of any initial decision to be the number of acceptable options at the planning horizon with which it is compatible, expressed as a ratio of the total number of acceptable options at the planning horizon.

The essence of the basic robustness approach is conveyed by Figure 5.2. This represents a problem in which there are three decision points. At the first decision point you can choose Options 2, 3, 4 or 5. Having chosen Option 2, for example, at the second decision point you can choose Options 6 or 7. And having chosen Option 6, at the 3rd decision point you can choose Options 15, 16, 17 or 22.

Each of the final Options 15 to 31 is rated under each of four scenarios. In this case Rosenhead has used a simple classification of desirable, acceptable, undesirable, catastrophic and questionable.

He suggests defining the *robustness* and *debility* of decision C1 given future F1 as

$$\text{robustness} = \frac{\text{number of acceptable options kept open, given decision C1 and future F1}}{\text{total number of acceptable options given F1}}$$

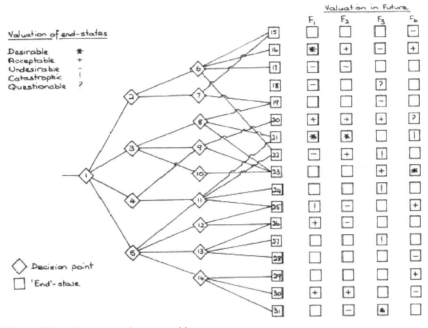

**Figure 5.2** A three-stage planning problem

Source: Rosenhead and Mingers (2001).

$$\text{and debility} = \frac{\text{number of unacceptable options still open, given decision C1 and future F1}}{\text{total number of unacceptable options given F1}}$$

He then suggests constructing robustness and debility matrices like Tables 5.7 and 5.8. These look a bit like payoff matrices, with decisions as rows and futures as columns.

**Table 5.7** The robustness matrix

| Choice | F1 | F2 | F3 | F4 |
|--------|-----|-----|-----|-----|
| 2 | 1/5 | 2/5 | 0/3 | 1/4 |
| 3 | 2/5 | 2/5 | 2/3 | 1/4 |
| 4 | 2/5 | 3/5 | 2/3 | 2/4 |
| 5 | 3/5 | 3/5 | 1/3 | 2/4 |

**Table 5.8** The debility matrix

| Choice | F1 | F2 | F3 | F4 |
|--------|-----|-----|-----|-----|
| 2 | 2/4 | 1/4 | 3/5 | 1/4 |
| 3 | 0 | 0 | 1/5 | 1/4 |
| 4 | 2/4 | 1/4 | 2/5 | 1/4 |
| 5 | 2/4 | 3/4 | 3/5 | 3/4 |

This use of a combination of indicators is a recurring theme in decision making. It echoes Roy's concordance and discordance indices, and the maximax and maximin criteria in game theory, and plays to decision makers' dual concerns: to grasp opportunities for very good outcomes and to avoid very bad ones. In this case, decision 2 seems poor in terms of robustness. Decisions 4 and 5 seem slightly better than decision 3. In terms of debility, decision 3 is clearly least bad.

Rosenhead offers no prescription for resolving the kind of trade-off that has arisen here. He describes robustness analysis as a format for exploring certain aspects of planning problems under uncertainty, rather than a method for finding an answer. Some of the types of structured information which participants may hope to have by the time they bring the process to an end are:

- a shortlist of possible decision packages rated in terms of their robustness against a variety of futures;
- a prediction of the shorter-term performance improvement to be expected from implementing each of the decision packages;
- some guidelines as to what actions by other interests linked to the planning process would be more or less beneficial; these can serve as the basis for contingency plans, or for incentives to encourage mutually advantageous behaviour;
- an assessment of which of the alternative futures the system, given its current condition and evolution, is particularly vulnerable to; this can focus lobbying or opinion-forming efforts on trying to influence the occurrence of futures which, in the light of current strategies, would present particular threats or opportunities.

## Linked decisions and strategic choice

Now consider uncertainty of a quite different kind. Friend (2001) distinguishes between three types:

 **Uncertainties**

*Uncertainties pertaining to the working Environment: UE for short*

This is the kind of uncertainty that can be dealt with by responses of a relatively *technical* nature: by surveys, research investigations, forecasting exercises, costing estimations. The response can range from an informal telephone conversation with an expert at one extreme, to the initiation of an elaborate exercise in mathematical modelling at the other.

The type of concern which this response reflects is generally of the form: 'This decision is difficult because we don't know enough about its circumstances, because we can't readily predict what the consequences of different ways forward might be.'

*Uncertainties pertaining to guiding Values: UV for short*

This is the kind of uncertainty which calls for a more *political* response. This response might take various forms – a request for policy guidance from a higher authority, an exercise to clarify objectives, a programme of consultations among affected interests. Again, the level of response may vary from the most informal of soundings to the most elaborate exercise for involving interest groups in the evaluation of alternative proposals.

Here, the concern on the part of the decision makers tends to take the form: 'This decision is difficult for us because there are so many conflicting objectives, priorities, interests . . ., because we don't have a clear enough view of where we should be going.'

*Uncertainties pertaining to related agendas: UR for short*

This is the kind of uncertainty that calls for a response in the form of exploration of the *structural* relationships between the decision currently in view and others with which it appears to be interconnected. The call here may be to expand the agenda of decision, to negotiate or collaborate with other decision makers, to move to a broader planning perspective – for the more linked decisions are to be considered, the more likely it becomes that time horizons will lengthen, and that some at least of the decisions will be 'owned' by other people. Again, the level of response may vary from the most informal exploration across organizational boundaries to the most formal planning exercise.

The concern on the part of decision makers here tends to take the form: 'This decision is difficult because we have been viewing it in too restricted terms, because we can't treat it in isolation from . . .'

So far in this chapter you have been concerned primarily with uncertainty about what will happen – what Friend calls UE. His UV – uncertainty because people disagree about what is good – was touched upon in Chapter 1 and taken further in Chapters 3 and 4. In the remainder of this chapter you will be concerned with UR. This is uncertainty about where the boundaries of the decision problem should lie. It can be tempting to think that a situation is hopelessly complex, everything is connected to everything else, and the only practical thing to do is ignore the bigger picture and tinker in isolation.

Friend has proposed a whole methodology for addressing uncertainty in decision making, which he has called the Strategic Choice approach. His method for approaching uncertainty around related decision fields, which he calls Analysis of Interconnected Decision Areas or AIDA, is only one part of this, but perhaps the most distinctive part.

A *decision area* is 'any area of choice within which decision makers can conceive of alternative courses of action that might be adopted, now or at some future time' (Friend 2001). This concept is fundamental to the approach. The first task for AIDA is to identify the distinct decision areas in a problem, the links between them and the priorities attached to them.

## ✐ Activity 5.4

Suppose you are a member of the management team of a district hospital. The team has identified a number of decisions that need to be made relating to the development of the hospital and the services it provides, and the implications of taking each option forward.

Currently the key decision is whether to become an independent organization or to remain under the management of the Ministry of Health (MoH). This decision is urgent as it has major implications for the strategic development of the hospital but it would need a considerable input from management to draw up a proposal which meets the requirements for independence set by government. The managers have decided that one essential for independence is a new information technology system to provide better information on treatment costs, and this would have major implications for the equipment budget. Another essential to becoming independent is improvement in the efficiency of the services offered. The hospital would have to develop a day surgery unit of 10 dedicated beds and buy new surgical equipment. The expected increase in demand for day surgery will cause a problem for patients with parking their cars unless additional space is provided for this. There would be substantial demands on the hospital's capital budget.

On the other hand, if the hospital remains a managed unit under the supervision of the MoH, the hospital would be required by the MoH to introduce medical audit. This would involve substantial amounts of management time and additional spending on information technology.

The Board is also considering two other important strategic options:

1   Because of its position near the motorway, the hospital could develop a trauma centre. This would involve setting up a neurosurgery unit. Such a unit would have major budget implications for staffing, equipment and capital budgets, and the Ministry of Health is against it. Thus the trauma centre can only be developed if the hospital becomes independent, and the work could not start until next year.
2   The hospital runs a psychiatric department which is separated from the main site in an old building. It is seen as important to improve the conditions in this department and there are plans to bring the psychiatric services on to the main site. Building a new psychiatric wing has major capital budget implications but it is expected that the sale of the old site will release some funds for this.

The finance department has calculated that because of limits on the capital available to them, a trauma centre and a new psychiatric wing could not be started in the same year. Also there is not enough space to build both a new psychiatric wing and a car park for the day surgery.

The management board wants to evaluate its options in a systematic way and has asked you to help. Identify the decision areas from the above case study. List the key factors that need to be considered in each area and note its level of importance or urgency.

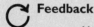

**Feedback**

You should have identified the areas listed in Table 5.9. The order of the list is unimportant. If your list looks somewhat different, go back and check that there are no differences of any substance.

**Table 5.9** Key decision areas, linking factors and priority levels

*Decision area*

1 Seek independent status
   - management time
   - priority: *urgent*
2 Provide better information on treatment costs
   - computer hardware/software: equipment budget implications
   - essential for gaining independent trust status
3 Develop day surgery
   - surgical equipment, 10 dedicated beds: budget implications
   - problems unless parking space provided
   - essential to becoming a trust
4 Introduce medical audit
   - management time
   - computer and software: budget implications
   - required if remaining directly managed by MoH
5 Develop trauma centre
   - introduce neurosurgery
   - employ staff and buy equipment: budget implications
   - MoH against it: cannot be done unless independent
   - priority: *important*
6 Bring psychiatric services on site in new wing
   - may release capital from sale of old site
   - major capital budget implications
   - would occupy space for day surgery car park
   - priority: *important*

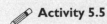 **Activity 5.5**

The next step is to draw a *decision graph*. First, set out the six decision areas as labelled circles or ellipses, spread out over a piece of paper. Then add more detail, using the following conventions suggested by Friend:

- If two decision areas are directly linked (i.e. the feasibility or desirability of options in area A is affected by the choice of options in area B), draw a line between them.
- If the link is weak or doubtful, show it with a broken or dotted line.
- If a decision area is urgent, put a dotted or shaded fringe around it.
- If a decision is important, put a double line around it.

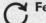 **Feedback**

Your diagram should look something like Figure 5.3. For clarity, the reasons for the links have been shown, but this is not really essential. In this example only six decision areas were involved. Reality can be even more complex and you will probably have to try different arrangements of the decision areas to avoid links running across each other as far as possible. This will also help you identify isolated and closely interconnected clusters.

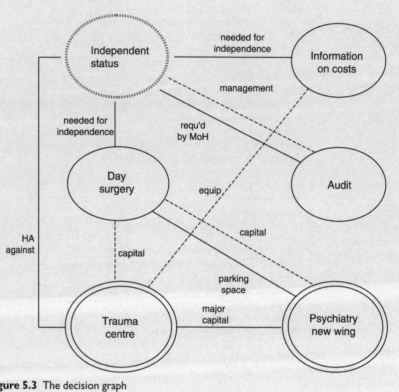

**Figure 5.3** The decision graph
Source: LSHTM.

---

### Activity 5.6

The next step is to identify the options that connect decision areas by assessing their mutual compatibility. The key tool here is the *option graph*, a development of the decision graph. This will help you to build the *option tree* of mutually compatible schemes.

First, extend Table 5.9 by adding another column that shows the options for each decision area. Mostly in this case they will be 'yes' or 'no'.

Second, draw a new version of the decision graph. It is a good idea to simplify it if possible at this stage by leaving out some of the decision areas that are expected to be less important and/or less connected to the important ones. For this exercise, you should aim to focus on four decision areas. For example, medical audit is less inter-connected than other areas. You may be planning to introduce audit anyway but if not, you could treat it as part of the decision on going independent.

Represent the options in each decision area and the links between *incompatible* ones in the way shown in Figure 5.4. These links are called *option bars*. (You could link compatible options instead but usually there are fewer incompatible options than compatible ones and so this way the diagram is less confusing. If you are not sure whether two options are incompatible, use a dotted option bar.)

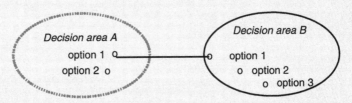

**Figure 5.4** Elements of the option graph

## Feedback

In this case study there are up to three options within each decision area, shown in Table 5.10. Your option graph should look something like Figure 5.5. For example, the

**Table 5.10** The options for each decision area

| Decision area | Options |
|---|---|
| 1 Seek independent (trust) status | yes/no |
| 2 Better information on treatment costs | yes/no |
| 3 Develop day surgery | with car park/without/no |
| 4 Introduce medical audit | yes/no |
| 5 Develop trauma centre | start next year/no |
| 6 Bring psychiatric services on site in new wing | start this year/next year/no |

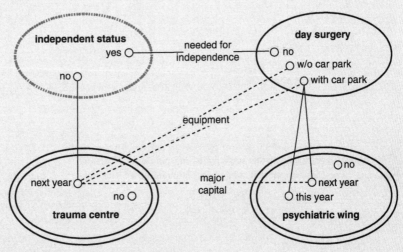

**Figure 5.5** Option graph for district hospital

solid line between 'no' to day surgery and 'yes' to independent status means that this combination is incompatible; day surgery is essential to independent status. The dotted lines indicate a less rigid link; day surgery and the trauma centre are in competition for a limited equipment budget but it may be possible to negotiate an increase in this budget if necessary.

## Activity 5.7

The last task is to represent all the compatible options in the four decision areas in Figure 5.5 in an *option tree*. A start has been made on the construction of the option tree in Figure 5.6. By convention, 'X' represents an option bar, i.e. an infeasible option or branch of the tree. ('?' represents dotted option bars.) Thus according to this part of the tree, independent status with day surgery plus parking and a trauma centre next year is incompatible with a new psychiatric wing. This is because the site is being used for the day surgery car park. Also next year's capital allocation is being used for the trauma centre. You have to complete the branches of the tree indicated by dotted lines.

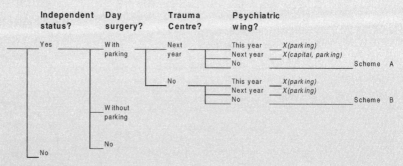

**Figure 5.6** Constructing an option tree

## Feedback

The completed option tree should look something like Figure 5.7. The sequence of branches is unimportant but the list of 14 compatible schemes should be the same. For each X, the reason for the bar is given in brackets.

What the analysis of interconnected decision areas (AIDA) has done is to produce a systematic listing of the range of feasible decision schemes. These can then be shortlisted and compared using methods such as those suggested in Chapter 4.

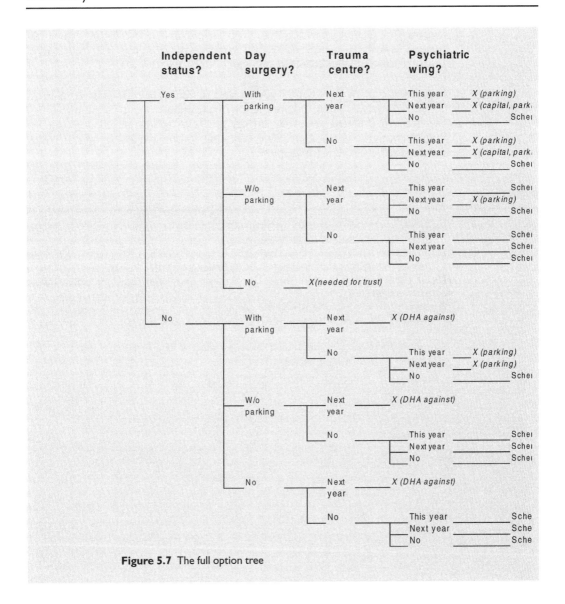

**Figure 5.7** The full option tree

## Summary

In this chapter you have learned about decision making where there is uncertainty. You have learned about three kinds of uncertainty: about outcomes, about values and about the boundaries of the decision problem.

You have learned about two approaches to dealing with uncertainty about outcomes: game theory and robustness analysis. In terms of game theory, you learned about three strategies: maximax, maximin and minimax regret, and how the approach adopted by a decision maker will depend on his or her attitude to risk. In robustness analysis you learned about the trumpet of uncertainty and indicators of the robustness and debility of the different options at each stage.

In the last part of the chapter you learned about AIDA, the analysis of interconnected decision areas. Where there was uncertainty about the boundaries of the decision problem you drew up decision and option graphs showing the links between the decision areas involved, and constructed an option tree which provided a shortlist of feasible options.

## References

Daellenbach H (2002) Uncertainty, in H Daellenbach and RL Flood *The Informed Student Guide to Management Science*. London: Thomson.

Friend J (2001) The Strategic Choice approach, in Rosenhead J and Mingers J (eds) *Rational Analysis for a Problematic World Revisited*. Chichester: John Wiley & Sons.

Friend J and Hickling A (eds) (2004) *The Strategic Choice Approach* (3rd edn). Oxford: Architectural Press.

Rosenhead J (2001) Robustness Analysis: keeping your options open, in Rosenhead J and Mingers J (eds) *Rational Analysis for a Problematic World Revisited*. Chichester: John Wiley & Sons.

Rosenhead J and Mingers J (eds) (2001) *Rational Analysis for a Problematic World Revisited*. Chichester: John Wiley & Sons, Ltd.

## Overview

In this chapter you will learn about an approach to decision making called Decision Analysis (note the capital letters) that is based on estimates of the probabilities of each state of nature. It is also based on measures of the overall desirability of each outcome, called its utility, so ultimately it is a one-criterion approach. The structure of the decision making problem is represented as a decision tree. You will examine the sensitivity of decisions to different assumptions about the probabilities involved. Finally, there is a brief introduction to decision conferencing, in which Decision Analysis is used by groups.

## Learning objectives

**By the end of this chapter, you will be better able to:**

- **represent the structure of a decision making problem as a decision tree**
- **calculate the expected utility of different decision options**
- **carry out a sensitivity analysis based on a decision tree**
- **describe the method of decision conferencing for group decision making**

## Key terms

**Chance node** A point at which a decision tree branches into a mutually exclusive set of states of nature. A chance node is usually represented by a circle.

**Decision Analysis** An approach to decision making which involves representing the problem in decision-tree form, branching at decision nodes and chance nodes. Probabilities are needed for each branch out of a chance node and utilities for each final branch in the tree.

**Decision node** The point in a decision tree where a decision must be made between competing and mutually exclusive policy or treatment options.

**Decision tree** A type of model of a decision making problem with branches representing the possible decision options and states of nature.

**Expected utility** The benefit or satisfaction that an individual anticipates getting from consuming a particular good or service.

**Lottery** A hypothetical gamble used in Decision Analysis to estimate the utility of an outcome.

**Decision outcome** A combination of decision options and states of nature. Each 'terminal' branch of the decision tree represents an outcome.

> **Utility** Happiness or satisfaction a person gains from consuming a commodity.

## What is a decision tree?

A decision tree is a type of model of a decision problem. An example from clinical decision making (whether to carry out a radical hysterectomy or not) is given in Figure 6.1 (Thornton et al. 1992). (Ignore the four figures in bold for the moment.)

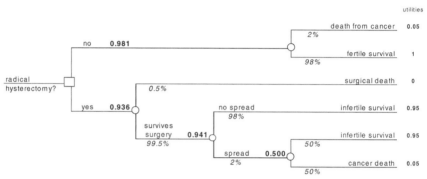

**Figure 6.1** A decision tree

Source: Adapted from Thornton et al. (1992).

It is constructed according to the following conventions:

1  Imagine a tree lying on its side, with its trunk on the left repeatedly subdividing into branches as you move to the right. The trunk represents the first (and sometimes the only) decision point. The tree finishes with the terminal branches on the right, which represent the full set of different possible *outcomes* (combinations of decision options and states of nature).
2  Each subdivision of the tree represents either a *decision node* (usually represented as a square) or a *chance node* (usually represented by a circle).
3  Branches from a decision node represent the mutually exclusive and exhaustive set of possible decision options at that point.
4  Branches leading out of a chance node represent the states of nature that could occur after going down the branch leading in to the node. After taking the 'no radical mastectomy' branch in Figure 6.1, the patient may or may not die of cancer. Each branch is labelled with the *probability* of the state of nature in question actually occurring. The branches leading out of a chance node are a mutually exclusive and exhaustive set of outcomes, and so the sum of their probabilities must add up to 1.0.
5  Each terminal branch is labelled with a *utility* (or disutility). This indicates the payoff associated with the outcome represented.

The data required are the same as for the approach to decision making under uncertainty described in Chapter 5, except that probabilities of each state of nature are also needed. These will have to be estimated. The payoffs or utilities will also have to be estimated. Decision Analysis is associated with a particular approach to this, known as the standard gamble.

In Figure 6.1 there is only one decision node, at the far left of the tree: whether the patient should have a radical hysterectomy or not. At each chance node the probability of taking each branch is given in italics. Probabilities are shown as percentages to help distinguish them from utilities. If the patient does not have the operation, the risk of death from cancer is 2 per cent but she preserves her fertility.

If she *does* have the operation there is a small (0.5 per cent) risk of death as a result of surgery. If she survives surgery, she will be infertile and there is still a 2 per cent chance of the cancer spreading, followed by a 50 per cent chance of death from cancer. However, the far more likely outcome (98 per cent) is that the cancer does not spread and she survives but is infertile.

You can work out the risk of death if she chooses surgery as follows: it is 0.5 per cent (due to surgical death) plus 99.5 per cent × 2 per cent × 50 per cent (the probability of surviving the operation *and* the cancer spreading *and* the cancer proving fatal). This is 0.5 per cent + 1 per cent or 1.5 per cent, which is better than the risk of death of 2 per cent if she does not have the operation.

Now read the following extract from Thornton and colleagues (1992). (Distal means furthest away from the core, as in distal finger joints. Proximal means near, or one step nearer to the core.)

 **Decision Analysis in medicine**

This does not, however, mean that radical hysterectomy is the best treatment because we have not considered all the relevant factors, for example, the patient's preference for delayed death from cancer versus immediate death from surgery, the desire to avoid the morbidity of surgery, and above all the desire to conserve fertility. We need to measure outcomes in a way that will allow us to see what chance of one favoured outcome our patient will relinquish to obtain another favoured outcome. When we have such a measure we can combine these utilities with the probabilities in a logical fashion to calculate the treatment with the highest expected utility.

The best method for measuring people's utilities is the basic reference lottery where the relative utilities of three health states are worked out together. Our patient needed to define the utility of four health states so two lotteries were needed. She ranked the health states as follows: the best was fertile life (with a utility of 1), the worst immediate death (with a utility of 0), with infertile life and delayed death rated intermediate. She did not find it difficult to rank infertile life as preferable to delayed death, but she also needed to know exactly where to place the intermediate states on her utility scale.

She first calculated the utility of infertile life by choosing between that and various gambles between fertile life and immediate death until she reached a level of indifference. It worked as follows. She was asked to imagine two doors, through one of which she had to go. Behind the left-hand door there was no risk of death but she would be rendered infertile. Behind the right-hand door she would encounter a 50 per cent chance of fertile survival but also a 50 per cent risk of death. She chose the left-hand door. The risks of death through the right-hand door were decreased until a point was reached where she could not decide which door to select. This occurred when the risk of death through the right-hand door was 5 per cent and of fertile survival 95 per cent. This was the level of indifference. Our patient therefore valued survival with infertility as 0.95 on a scale where full health was valued 1 and immediate death valued 0. She performed a second similar lottery between delayed death from cancer and various chances of full health or immediate death and derived a utility for delayed death of 0.05.

There are alternative methods of measuring values, such as asking patients to mark health states on a linear scale, but, unlike the reference gamble, this method is not axiomatically correct. People avoid the extremes of the scale, and because they may not perceive the trade-off inherent in the technique, the values obtained in this way may be distorted. A better alternative makes use of natural underlying scales such as money or years of life. Unfortunately people's utilities for money and years of life are rarely linear. People are usually risk-seeking or risk-averse. For example, the gambler in our earlier example is likely to be risk-seeking.

Having measured the utilities we need to combine them with the probabilities to select a preferred course of action – that is, that with the greatest *expected utility*. We start by estimating the utility of each chance node, which is calculated as the weighted average of the utilities of its possible outcomes, where the weights are the probabilities of each outcome. The utility of the upper chance node in Figure 6.1 is thus $(2\% \times 0.05) + (98\% \times 1.0) = 0.981$. Where there is a sequence of chance nodes in the tree we use the weighted utility of the distal chance node in calculating the expected utility of the proximal node. The utility of a decision node is the maximum of the utilities of its component branches since a rational decision maker should choose this strategy. It is clear that the expected utility of no further surgery (0.981) is greater than that of radical hysterectomy (0.936), and this is the option our patient should choose.

The difference in expected utility between the different courses of action may not appear very great, but on this scale the difference 0.045 represents 4–5 per cent of the value of the patient's entire life in full health. Moreover, if the axioms of expected utility theory are accepted by our patient (most people do agree that this is how they wish to make decisions), and if the probability and value estimates are the best possible, then it would be perverse to choose the course of lower utility, however small the difference.

The final part of a full decision analysis should include a sensitivity analysis, because conclusions depend on the probabilities and utilities used, and in real life we are rarely, if ever, certain what these are. In a sensitivity analysis each of the key probabilities and values is varied in turn within the range of reasonable uncertainty to test the robustness of the conclusion. Figure 6.2 presents a one-way sensitivity analysis to show the effect of varying the utility of infertility. Each straight line on the graph represents the expected utility of the relevant strategy at a range of levels of infertility utility. The strategy lines intersect at an infertility utility of 0.995; therefore, above this value radical surgery is the preferred option while below it no further surgery is preferred. The point at which strategy lines intersect is called a decision threshold. This threshold will itself vary if other variables such as operative mortality and recurrence risk are changed.

The effect of changing more than one variable can be shown in a threshold analysis (Figure 6.3). Here the decision threshold is plotted against the risk of recurrence and utility of infertility for three different operative death rates [one line for each]. For each patient the utility of infertility and probability of disease spread are plotted. If this point falls below and

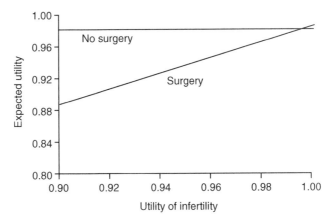

**Figure 6.2** Sensitivity analysis

Source: Thornton et al. (1992).

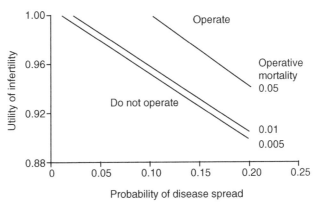

**Figure 6.3** Threshold analysis

Source: Thornton et al. (1992).

to the left of the relevant threshold line, she should not undergo surgery and if above and to the right, she should. The effect of varying utilities and probabilities can be seen at a glance. Decision trees and sensitivity and threshold analyses can easily become complicated and so computerised aids are widely used by serious practitioners.

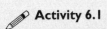 **Activity 6.1**

In Figure 6.1, how was the expected utility of the lower branch (0.936) calculated?

**Feedback**

The lower branch divides at the chance nodes indicated by the circles into a series of sub-branches. Although when you are drawing up the tree you usually work from left to right, when calculating expected utilities you work from right to left. This is known as folding back the decision tree.

First consider the right-hand chance node on the lower branch. This is associated with two scenarios:

• the *infertile survival* branch; this has probability 50 per cent and utility 0.95, so the contribution of this branch to the expected utility of being at this (right-hand) chance node is (50% * 0.95) = 0.475

• the *death from cancer* branch; this has probability 50 per cent and utility 0.05, so the contribution of this branch is (50% * 0.05) = 0.025.

Thus the expected utility of the right-hand node (and therefore of the branch leading to it called 'spread') is 0.475 + 0.025 = 0.5, as shown in Figure 6.1.

Now consider the next node to the left, which splits into 'no spread' and 'spread':

• in this case the *no spread* branch leads to infertile survival, with probability 98 per cent and utility 0.95; the contribution of this branch to the expected utility of being at this chance node is (98% * 0.95) = 0.931

• the *spread* branch has probability 2 per cent and, as you have just calculated, an expected utility of 0.5; the contribution of this branch is thus (2% * 0.5) = 0.01.

Thus the expected utility of the no spread/spread node is 0.941.

Similarly, you may calculate the expected utility of the next chance node to the left (*surgical death/survival*) as:

• surgical death = 0.5% * 0.0 = 0.0

• survival = 99.5% * 0.941 = 0.936.

The implication of this is that the patient should choose *no further surgery* as this has a higher expected utility (0.981) than choosing radical hysterectomy (0.936).

Remember that this procedure for calculating the expected utility is only appropriate for chance nodes. At a decision node in the body of the tree, you assume that the branch with the highest expected utility will be chosen. This means that the expected utility of a decision node is the maximum of the expected utilities of branches out of it.

 **Activity 6.2**

What problems can you see in the practical application of Decision Analysis to a management problem as opposed to a clinical one?

**Feedback**

One key factor is that many *clinical* decision problems are variations on a theme. The question of whether or not someone should have a hysterectomy, for example, is one that comes up for many different women. As a result, it is possible to develop standard decision trees for a number of common problems and there are data in the research literature on many of the probabilities involved. The tasks for any specific Decision Analysis are then limited to two options:

1 Revise the standard probabilities in the light of particular characteristics of the patient.

2 Establish the patient's utilities.

By contrast, many *management* decisions are 'one-off'. A new tree may have to be developed for each problem and there may be very little in the way of data or direct experience on which to base estimates of probability.

Another distinction lies in the roles of the parties involved in the decision. In the clinical context there is a clear contrast between:

• the professional, who has the technical knowledge of the different outcomes and so supplies the structure of the tree and the probabilities;
• the patient, whose life will be affected and so should be the source of the utilities, which embody factors such as attitudes to risk, pain and disability.

One of the advantages of Decision Analysis in a clinical context is that it can clarify this distinction and ensure that patients' utilities influence decisions. In *management* decisions, however, a number of decision makers may have differing but equally legitimate, assessments of the probabilities and utilities involved. *Sensitivity analysis* may be able to show that some of these differences of opinion would have little impact on the best decision and focus attention on where better data are worth obtaining or differences of opinion have to be resolved. With goodwill, the result can be better understanding of the problem and a well-informed consensus but this may require skilful facilitation.

## A decision tree in health services management

In Chapter 5 you used game theory to analyse how far to extend the main operating theatre block of an acute hospital. Now you will use a decision tree for the same problem. On your CD there is a file called 'Ch6DecTree'. This includes a spreadsheet called 'Tree' which shows the branching structure.

After discussions with managers at the neighbouring hospital and with local surgeons, your management group has decided that it is possible to estimate the probabilities of the different scenarios involved, as follows:

• that the neighbouring hospital will expand: 60 per cent
• that the day surgery report will be generally accepted: 40 per cent.

You also need the utilities of each outcome. Use the absolute differences between capacity and expected demand, in the same way as in Activity 5.2. Note that the layout in the decision tree assumes that the two events that make up the state of nature in this problem (expansion of neighbour and acceptance of report) are unrelated or independent. This means that:

- the problem can be represented by two successive chance nodes on each branch from the decision node, one for each event;
- the order of the chance nodes on each decision node branch does not matter; the split between 'neighbour builds/doesn't build' event could just as well have been after the split between the 'report accepted/not accepted' event.

If events were *not* independent, the tree would be drawn with only one chance node in each decision branch and four branches from it, each representing a combination of events.

In this example, standard spreadsheet software was used to create the tree by formatting the borders of cells and using the drawing tools for the squares and circles at the nodes. Alternatively you could rely entirely on the drawing tools. You can reduce the amount of formatting and typing in of formulae that you have to do when you are drawing replicated branches by using the copy and paste commands.

 **Activity 6.3**

Using your spreadsheet software, and the probabilities and utilities that you have been given, calculate expected utilities for each (non-terminal) branch of the tree. Show on the decision tree the probabilities and expected utilities for each branch. How many new theatres should you build, using these 'baseline' assumptions?

 **Feedback**

A completed tree is given in the spreadsheet 'Tree 2' in 'Ch6DecTree'. You can see the formulae involved for one branch in the spreadsheet called 'Formulae'. In this workbook, data and calculations are on separate worksheets, 'Tree 2' and 'Tables' respectively. This is often recommended as good spreadsheet practice.

Notice how the probabilities in 'Tree 2' are taken from cells C3 and C4 in 'Tables', by prefixing the cell reference with the name of the worksheet. The *expected* utilities are the sum of the probability * expected utility for each branch. For example, the expected utility of being on the 'neighbour builds' arm if you decide to build 0 is = 'Tables'!C$4*F5 + (1−'Tables'!C$4)*F8.

Working backwards through the tree, you should have found that the option with the smallest 'expected disutility' is to build one, for which the expected utility is −1.72. This is better than −2.04 for build none and −2.44 for build two.

For a more complicated tree you might consider using more specialized Decision Analysis software, which does much of the work in setting up the tree and analysing it for you.

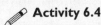 **Activity 6.4**

Some members of your group of decision makers disagree about the estimates of probability. How sensitive are your results to the probability estimates of 40 per cent and 60 per cent?

To answer this, construct two tables with:

- hypothetical values of probability from 0 to 1 as the rows (with, say, intervals of 0.1 thus: 0.0, 0.1, 0.2, etc.);
- the three decision options as the columns;
- expected utilities in the cells.

The first table should show how the expected utilities of each decision option vary with the probability that the day surgery report will be accepted. To guide you, a skeleton version is provided (Table 6.1). Note that for this sensitivity analysis, the probability of the neighbouring hospital expanding has been fixed at its 'central' value of 0.6.

**Table 6.1** Skeleton table for sensitivity analysis

| Sensitivity to assumption about acceptance of report Assumption: $p(neighbour\ expands) = 0.6$ | | |
| --- | --- | --- |
| p(report) | build 0 | build 1 | build 2 |
| 0.0 | | | |
| 0.1 | | | |
| 0.2 | | | |
| 0.3 | | | |
| 0.4 | | | |
| 0.5 | | | |
| 0.6 | | | |
| 0.7 | | | |
| 0.8 | | | |
| 0.9 | | | |
| 1.0 | | | |

Your second table should show how the expected utilities of each decision option vary with the probability that the neighbouring hospital will expand, with the probability that the day surgery report will be generally accepted fixed at its central value of 0.4.

 **Feedback**

The spreadsheet 'Tables' on 'Ch6DecTree' gives completed tables for the sensitivity analyses and shows two ways of constructing them.

### Register/'paste special' method

The first way involves creating a register, shown in the range A6:D8. Note that B8:D8 contain copies of the expected utilities of each option from the tree in 'Tree+'.

Place the value 0 in C4 and see what happens in the register cells B8:D8. These are the expected utilities of the three options for $p$(expand) = 0.6 and $p$(accept) = 0. Copy B8:D8 by value into the range B19:D19. (Look back at Chapter 2 if you have forgotten how to copy values.)

Now place the value 0.1 in C4 and copy B8:D8 by value into B20:D20. Continue in this way until you have completed the table.

Build up Table S2 in a similar way but changing the values in C3 rather than C4.

### Formula method

A second method of constructing these tables is also shown in 'Tables' in rows 33 to 58. The first step is to create a single formula for the expected utility of branch 1 (build none) and place it in B48.

If p is prob(neighbour expands), q is prob(report accepted) and u1 to u4 are the utilities at the ends of the branches for 'build 0', the formula is

$$p*(q*u01 + (1-q)*u02) + (1-p)*(q*u03 + (1-q)*u04)$$

But for this formula you must take the probability q of acceptance of the report not from \$C\$4, but from the range A48. You can then copy this formula down the column and it will automatically incorporate the range of probabilities in A48:A58.

The problem with this method is that a formula like this can become very long and complicated and it is easy to make mistakes. Once you have got the formula right though, it is very quick to copy and you have the great advantage of a dynamic table: one that changes automatically as you make changes to the utilities, for example.

 **Activity 6.5**

Use your spreadsheet software to produce two line charts showing the sensitivity of the expected utility of each option to estimated probabilities, one from your Table 6.1a and one from your Table 6.2a in 'Tables'.

 **Feedback**

A chart based on Table 6.1a in 'Tables', showing the sensitivity of the expected utility of each option to different probabilities that the report will be accepted, is shown in 'Ch6DecTree' as 'SA p report accepted'. You can see that 'build 1' is the best option for all probabilities between 0 and about 67 per cent if the other assumptions remain unaltered.

Figure 6.4 shows the sensitivity of the expected utility of each option to different probabilities that the neighbours will expand. This shows that 'build 1' is the best option for all probabilities between about 40 per cent and about 70 per cent if the other assumptions remain unaltered. Below 40%, 'build 0' is best and above 70%, 'build 2' is best.

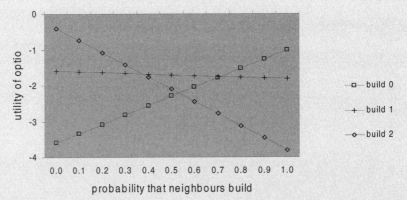

**Figure 6.4** Sensitivity analysis on probability that neighbour will expand

This type of analysis is called a one-way sensitivity analysis because only one datum is varied while other data are fixed. You can also do two-way sensitivity analyses. The tables in A61:L102 in 'Tables' show, for each option, how expected utility varies with different combinations of p(neighbour expands) and p(report accepted). This suggests what is known as a threshold analysis. Using the formula in the feedback to Activity 6.4, the expected utilities are as follows:

For   'build 0':  $p*(q*u01 + (1 - q)*u02) + (1 - p)*(q*u03 + (1 - q)*u04)$
      'build 1':  $p*(q*u11 + (1 - q)*u12) + (1 - p)*(q*u13 + (1 - q)*u14)$

If you replace all the utilities in these expressions (u01, u02, etc. up to u14) with the values in the tree ($-1, -1$, etc. up to $-2$), the expected utilities reduce to the following:

      'build 0':  $3p - pq + q - 4$
      'build 1':  $p - 3pq + q - 2$

At the threshold or borderline between 'build 0' and 'build 1', the expected utilities of these two options are the same, i.e. $3p - pq + q - 4 = p - 3pq + q - 2$.

After some algebra this reduces to $q = 1/p - 1$, and you can use this expression to plot the 'threshold' line which separates the 'build 0' area from the 'build 1' area.

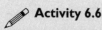

**Activity 6.6**

Using a method similar to the above, derive an expression for the threshold line between 'build 1' and 'build 2'.

**Feedback**

From the feedback to Activity 6.5 for 'build 1', the formula in the feedback to Activity 6.4 for 'build 2', and the utility values in the tree for u11 to u14, you have:

        'build 1':    $p - 3pq + q - 2$

and    'build 2':    $p*(q*u21 + (1 - q)*u22) + (1 - p)*(q*u23 + (1 - q)*u24)$

so using the utility values in the tree for u21 up to u24, you have

    build 2:    $-3p - pq - q$

At the threshold, the utility of 'build 1' is the same as the utility of 'build 2', so

    $p - 3pq + q - 2 = -3p - pq - q,$

and hence $p = (1 - q)/(2 - q)$

These two threshold lines are shown in Figure 6.5. For combinations of probabilities in the top right-hand corner of the diagram, you build none. In the bottom left-hand corner you build 2, and in the diagonal (light grey) band across the middle you build 1.

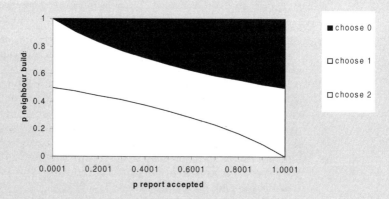

**Figure 6.5** Decision frontier analysis for both probabilities in the tree

Now you have completed an analysis very similar to that done by Thornton and colleagues, and which most people rely on specialist software to do for them.

## Multi-attribute utility analysis

Suppose the outcome at the end of a given branch is best represented by more than one attribute. In a clinical decision tree, for example, both mortality rate *and* a morbidity rate might be important. To use the tree in the usual way, this would involve turning a multiple criteria problem into a single-criterion one by deriving a utility for each combination of attribute scores. Keeney and Raiffa (1976) developed a set of procedures for doing this, but multi-attribute utilities are difficult to obtain in practice. A more modest step is to use the tree to work out how the 'expected' scores for each attribute in turn vary for the different decision options (e.g. expected mortality rate and expected morbidity rate). The decision maker can then be offered a *set* of expected attribute scores for each decision option. However, this requires independence of preference assessments (see Chapter 4 again), and may not help if there are decision nodes in the middle of the tree, unless one branch dominates the others.

## Pros and cons of decision trees

Decision trees have a number of features, some of which can be either strengths or weaknesses, depending on the situation:

1 *Graphic representation*: the tree provides a model of the decision problem, with the advantages of providing an explicit basis for sharing knowledge and understanding of what is going on. However, the trees can quickly become very big and apparently complicated; large sub-trees may be duplicated many times. On a small scale, this duplication of sub-trees was a feature of the example you have just considered.

2 *Incorporates estimates of risk*: this is the key characteristic of the method, which is an advantage if there are reasonable estimates of risk available (as in a well-researched clinical problem) but arguably a disadvantage if there are not.

3 *Incorporates utilities*: the separation of risk and utility is one of the strong points of the method from a theoretical point of view. As you have seen, this has practical implications in clinical decision making when, in principle at least, the health care professional can supply the tree and the probabilities and the patient can supply the utilities. However, different methods of eliciting utilities can give different results and there may be questions about the validity and reliability of the values used. Also there are questions about what to do when there are many stakeholders with different utilities.

4 *Sensitivity analysis*: the fact that decision trees lend themselves readily to sensitivity analyses is a strength and in some circumstances can overcome concerns about the precision of the probability estimates and the validity of utilities. However, while one-dimensional sensitivity analyses are straightforward to conduct and interpret, the numbers of potential multi-dimensional analyses (which address the effect of varying more than one factor at a time) can become very large and the results difficult to present and understand.

5 *A single criterion approach*: in most examples of Decision Analysis in the literature the utility of each possible outcome is expressed as a single figure. The task is to choose the option that maximizes the expected value of this utility, so DA is

mainly used as a single-criterion decision method. As you saw in Chapter 4, many problems naturally involve more than one outcome criterion or attribute – morbidity as well as mortality for example.

## Decision conferencing

In Chapters 1 and 4 you came across the problem of different stakeholders having different values or different implicit models of the situation. Decision conferencing provides a controlled setting that helps to focus attention on achieving the decision making goal. The usual format is that computer-based Decision Analysis is used during a decision workshop to represent the different perspectives of the decision makers, to explore differences of opinion and to develop new and useful insights. The aim is not to tell the decision makers what to decide but rather to help them to understand their beliefs, judgements and preferences in the context of the choices facing them.

The process is typically supported by a facilitator and a decision analyst. The facilitator leads the workshop, guides the discussion and builds and interprets models of the decision making problem. The decision analyst handles the details of the model building.

An outline programme of a decision workshop could be as follows, although a two-day programme is not always practicable.

### Day 1

1  Formulate the problem.
2  Build the model.
3  Assess judgements, beliefs and the weights used to compare criteria.
4  Draw tentative conclusions.

### Day 2

1  Assess the results of the first day.
2  Revise and rebuild the model.
3  Perform a sensitivity analysis.
4  Draw conclusions and make recommendations.
5  Generate a plan of action and gain commitment.

In brief, the advantages of decision conferencing are that:

• All stakeholders have an opportunity to contribute and to share in the ownership of and responsibility for the resulting plan of action.
• It facilitates communication between decision makers by focusing on critical aspects of the decision making problem and avoiding non-productive debate of irrelevant issues.
• The knowledge and creativity brought to bear on the decision making problem are extended.
• Participants are able to reach a shared understanding of the nature of the

problem and the reasons for the decision, even if they do not all share the same priorities and utilities.

Its disadvantages are that:

- Like other methods of decision support, it is not productive in situations where the decision makers show little willingness to compromise and pursue a common interest.
- The time and cost involved make this method unsuitable for day-to-day management problems.

## Summary

In this chapter you have learnt how to structure a decision making problem using a decision tree. The tree contains data on probabilities (obtained from observation or subjective assessment) and utilities (obtained by using formal methods such as the standard gamble or consensus development). Decision options with the highest expected utility are found by folding back the tree.

You went on to construct tables for one-variable sensitivity analyses and expressions for two-variable threshold or 'frontier' analyses. Finally, you learnt how the methods of Decision Analysis are used in decision conferencing to facilitate consensus and build commitment among a group of decision makers.

## References

Inadomi JM (2004) Decision analysis and economic modeling: a primer. *European Journal of Gastroenterology and Hepatology* 16: 535–42.

Keeney RL and Raiffa H (1976) *Decisions with Multiple Objectives: Preferences and Value Trade-offs*. New York: Wiley.

Taylor BW (1999) Introduction to Management Science, in Taylor BW (ed.) *Decision Analysis and Game Theory*. Upper Saddle River, NJ: Prentice Hall.

Thornton JG, Lilford RJ and Johnson N (1992) Decision analysis in medicine. *British Medical Journal* 304: 1099–103.

## Further reading

Special issue of 1997; 17.

Detsky AS, Naglie G, Krahn MD, Naimark D and Redelmeier DA. Part 1: Getting Started, pp. 123–5.

Detsky AS, Naglie G, Krahn MD, Redelmeier DA and Naimark D. Part 2: Building a Tree, pp. 126–9.

Krahn MD, Naglie G, Naimark D, Redelmeier DA and Detsky AS. Part 4: Analyzing the Model and Interpreting the Results, pp. 142–51.

Naglie G, Krahn MD, Naimark D, Redelmeier DA and Detsky AS: Part 3: Estimating Probabilities and Utilities, pp. 136–41.

# SECTION 3

# Models for service planning and resource allocation

# 7 Population need for a specific service

## Overview

In this chapter you will learn about strategic intervention to ensure that health services are efficient and equitable. Among the tasks involved are estimating and forecasting the health care needs of populations, and ensuring that the existing configuration of services can meet these needs. A brief discussion of corporate needs assessment, in which an attempt is made to balance or resolve the various interest groups and pressures bearing on the service, is followed by a review of needs assessment based on a combination of data on the population served, evidence about the effectiveness and acceptability of treatment and explicit judgements about priorities, and the potential contribution to this of mathematical modelling.

## Learning objectives

By the end of this chapter, you will be better able to:

- explain the concept of need for health care and the implications for strategic intervention in publicly funded health care systems
- explain the role of needs assessment in strategic intervention
- describe the strengths and weaknesses of corporate needs assessment
- describe the strengths and weaknesses of a variety of approaches to population-based needs assessment, ranging from a crude norms-based approach to a full evidence-based approach

## Key terms

**Corporate needs assessment** A more or less formal process for adjusting the provision of health services in response to pressures for change from providers, central policy makers, professional bodies, patients and representatives of the public.

**Evidence-based needs assessment** A process through which the provision of health care can be responsive to the characteristics of the population served and evidence about the effectiveness and acceptability of the services in question.

**Population-based needs assessment** A process through which the provision of health care can be responsive to the characteristics of the population served.

**Population need for health** The gaps between actual and desired levels of health in a population.

---

**Population need for health care** The gaps between current levels of health in a population and the levels of health that they could enjoy if they had appropriate health care.

---

## Introduction: efficiency, equity, need and appropriateness

Planning implies objectives, in health care as in any other field of activity. What are the strategic objectives of a health care system? One easy answer is to improve health but you need to go a little deeper than this before you can address the question of how to meet health care needs.

### Efficiency

Given scarcity of resources, the people responsible for any system will be concerned with its efficiency – achieving the maximum output for a given level of inputs. Most health care systems now depend to a very substantial extent on public funding, whether through tax or social insurance. This has led to a concern on the part of many governments that the system that they are supporting should perform in a way that is consistent with their societal objectives. For this reason the outputs of health care systems are commonly seen as the health benefits they provide for the population (rather than, say, financial benefits for the system). If so, improving efficiency means increasing the health benefits produced by health care per unit cost.

### Equity

Efficiency is not the only criterion for a good system. Another objective in many societies is equity, or social justice, in the accessibility of health care to different groups within the population. More specific definitions of equity than this are a matter of debate. However, if we accept Whitehead's (1992) view of equity in health as 'fair opportunities for each individual to attain their full health potential, with no avoidable obstacles', it follows that the health care system should play its part in helping everyone achieve their full health potential and that the limited resources at its disposal should be used fairly. A degree of consensus has built around the ideas of

- *horizontal equity* people with equal need having equal access to health care; and
- *vertical equity* people with the greatest need having the highest priority.

Another societal objective is that health care should be humane – people (carers and staff as well as patients) should be treated with due consideration and respect – but this will not be addressed here as quantitative modelling has played very little part in its pursuit.

### Need

The pursuit of equity begs the question of what is meant by need. Thinking about how to plan health care led to efforts to clarify this. Two of the most useful contributions were from Culyer (1976), who distinguished between need for health and need for *health care*, and Matthew (1971), among others, who suggested that a need for health care existed when an individual had an illness or disability for which there was effective and acceptable treatment or care. An extension of Matthew's argument would imply that a need for health care exists only if an individual has a level of risk of illness or disability that can be reduced by acceptable care.

These contributions were important because they provided a clear link between equity and efficiency. If the outputs of the health care system are defined in terms of health benefits, and if the greater potential health benefit for someone, the greater their need for health care, then meeting greater needs *with the same inputs/ resources* will mean greater expected benefits. In these circumstances the pursuit of equity will also produce improvements in efficiency.

If this identification of need for care with potential to benefit is accepted, there are two key implications for any strategic analysis of population needs.

1  Assessment of need for health care involves information about expected benefits and harms, and the nature and extent of expected benefits and harms can only be assessed for *specific conditions and interventions*. These are matters for research and/or consensus development among technical experts.
2  Different people with different conditions can expect different types of benefit (for example, improvement of physical symptoms, improvement of mental symptoms, life extension, risk reduction) and objective assessment of the relative value of these different types of benefit is impossible. Planning or commissioning services involves *prioritization of benefits* and this involves value judgements. These are ultimately matters for the community or its representatives, although they may seek the advice of experts.

Some people are unhappy about his formulation, arguing that it medicalizes need. Certainly equity is widely interpreted as being about the elimination of differences in access to care between groups defined by their socio-economic status, ethnicity, or in some other way. The counter-argument is that as long as a person's access to care is dependent only on their potential to benefit, there will be equity between any set of population groups.

The difficulty arises if the same potential benefits cost more to realize in some groups than in others. For example, someone living in sub-standard housing may have a potential to benefit from health care that is similar to someone who is better off but it may cost more to achieve that benefit if, for example, day care is not a practical option for them. For the same reason, it may cost more to realize the full health potential of someone living a long way away from hospital than for someone living nearby. In this situation, efficiency gains mean equity losses, and a balance has to be struck between the two. Where this balance should lie is a matter for community and political judgement.

## Treatment decisions and appropriateness

At the time when the decision is made to treat a particular patient in a particular way, the outcome is often uncertain. Thus treatment decisions have to be made on the basis of predicted or expected benefits and harms. There may be relevant data from research studies but these are average results for groups of patients with particular attributes (specified diagnosis, no co-morbidity, etc.). In theory, these results provide initial estimates, which can then be modified by the clinical decision maker in the light of information about particular patients. Increasingly, treatment decisions are informed by *guidelines* based on research and consensus among experts, about what kind of treatment is appropriate for what kind of patient. These set out the indications (to ensure high enough expected benefit) and contra-indications (to ensure low enough expected harm) for treatment. To begin with, affordability was considered as a separate issue but increasingly a treatment option is only considered appropriate if there is an acceptable balance between expected benefits, harms and costs.

What happens if there is more than one appropriate treatment for a patient? In general, each option will involve a different balance of expected benefit, harm and cost. For example, surgery might involve greater risks of harm but greater possible benefits than medical treatment. As you learned in Chapter 6, many commentators think this is an ideal context for decision analysis, in which the technical or clinical expert supplies the probabilities and the patient supplies the values or utilities.

 **Activity 7.1**

1  What is the difference between health needs and health care needs?

2  In defining health care needs, what do you think are the respective roles of:

   (a)  experts such as doctors, other health care professionals and researchers
   (b)  patients
   (c)  the wider community?

 **Feedback**

1  Health needs are gaps between actual and desired levels of health. Health *care* needs (some people call them requirements) arise when people with health needs can expect benefit from health care. Note that:

   • health needs do not necessarily imply health care needs; but whether they do or not, they may also imply other kinds of intervention, particularly where risk reduction is required, such as health promotion and environmental controls;
   • improvements in the effectiveness of health care creates new or increased health care needs;
   • assessment of the relative need of a local population or group for a particular form of health care requires information on the amount of benefit its members can be expected to derive from it; and
   • comparing different types of need for care is difficult because comparing benefits is difficult; in general there is no *objectively* correct answer to the question of which local population or group has the greatest health care needs.

2  Needs assessment involves estimates of the types and probabilities of benefit and harm that can be expected as a result of intervention. Doctors and other experts are

the best source for these, informed by the results of research studies, meta-analyses and in the absence of these, expert consensus. It also involves prioritization of, and value judgements about, different types of benefit:

- In matters of choice between treatment options, these are matters for the patients concerned. (There may be different risks involved, for example.)
- In matters of priority between care programmes (the balance of funds to be spent on mental as opposed to physical health, for example) the community, or its representatives, should have a major role.

## Strategic intervention for equity and efficiency

If efficiency and equity are the main strategic aims of health care systems, a good health care system is one that moves as many people as possible out of the 'x' categories in Figure 7.1 and into the '✓' categories.

Balance of benefit, harms and costs

|  |  | Favourable | Unfavourable |
|---|---|---|---|
| Treatment provided | yes | met need for care ✓ | inappropriate use of health care × |
|  | no | unmet need for care × | no/low need for care, no use of it ✓ |

**Figure 7.1** Met and unmet need for care

What are the possible mechanisms for achieving this? One might be to leave it to the market, but markets for health care are very much less than perfect (and so do not produce efficiently). Very briefly, they do not provide for the following:

- consumer ignorance: most patients are unable to make informed judgements about appropriateness and it is unreasonable to expect otherwise;
- monopolistic providers;
- interventions with public benefits, e.g. immunization against infectious diseases, in which there are benefits for the unimmunized as a result of the general reduction in risk of infection;
- social concern for the health of others.

Health care markets are generally inequitable as well as inefficient because of the generally inverse relationship between capacity to benefit and capacity to pay, whether fees or insurance premiums.

The other *laissez-faire* option is to leave it to the providers. This would require clinical decision makers to do the following:

- ensure efficient and equitable use of the resources currently available to them by providing appropriate, cost-effective care for the patients most likely to benefit;
- seek to alter the levels and mix of resources available to them, if the current levels and mix are inconsistent with providing efficient and equitable care.

There is an increasing reluctance to rely on providers to do this on their own because:

- some medical specialties and health care providers are more influential than others;
- some patients are more clinically interesting than others;
- the wide local variations in rates of prescribing, hospital admission and elective surgery suggest that there are unexplained (and inequitable) variations between clinical decision makers in their practice.

If all this is accepted, the implication is that there is a need for strategic intervention. Clinical decisions have to be supported or constrained by the effects of strategic decisions (by managers, planners and policy makers), who ensure that systems are in place that support:

1 Good access, so that people with health care needs are offered appropriate care, through:

   (a) referral guidelines;
   (b) outreach and screening systems;
   (c) levels of activity and resources that are consistent with appropriate good quality care for the population served; and

2 Sound clinical decisions, through

   (a) treatment guidelines;
   (b) information and audit systems.

Behind all of these lies the economic and political environment, which will affect levels of health, roll-out and acceptance of technical and organizational change, the general levels of resources available, and the priority given to different objectives. Thus decision makers at local level will typically have to operate within the constraints and guidelines handed down from national levels.

## Approaches to health care needs assessment

Health care needs assessment is a systematic approach to item 1 (c) above: ensuring that the levels of activity and resources provided are consistent with equitable access to good quality care for the population served.

Here you will learn about two broad approaches to needs assessment: corporate and population-based. The *corporate* approach involves a process of adjustment subject to competing views and pressures. *Population-based* approaches take as their starting point data on the population served and involve different combinations of data, assumptions, calculation and judgement. The aim is to provide estimates of need which are independent of current local levels of supply with a view to identifying any major gaps between actual provision and what is 'needed'.

This is where model building comes in. After a brief review of corporate needs assessment, you will learn about these essentially quantitative approaches to determining the desired levels of activity and resources.

Note, though, that in practice, the levels of health care provided are inevitably the product of a 'corporate process'. Even when the most detailed population-based needs assessments are carried out, typically these will be used to inform the negotiations rather then determine their outcome.

## Corporate needs assessment

The most common approach to determining the mix of services provided to a given population is through a process of adjustment in response to pressures for change. These pressures may come from clinical decision makers and from central policy makers, professional bodies, patients and representatives of the public. The process of balancing interests and pressures has been called 'corporate needs assessment'. Although it may involve little actual assessment of needs, it does have a number of potential advantages:

- It is fairly close to what goes on in the absence of any attempt at rigorous analysis. It is possible to strengthen such processes by making them structured, open and transparent, and informed by data and analysis, rather than unaccountable and behind closed doors.
- It can be an incremental process (try a bit more here and a bit less there and see if that helps). The argument is that to improve equity and/or efficiency it is sufficient to identify the right direction to be moving at the current point in time, rather than the ideal or ultimate destination. This makes it less demanding of data and analysis than the population-based or 'zero-based' approaches.

The problems with this approach are that:

- decisions tend to be driven by negotiation, and hence by power relationships, rather than what is actually efficient or equitable;
- interested parties rarely press for fewer resources;
- the aspects of care that gain attention tend to be driven by events and crises, rather than leadership based on strategic objectives or anticipation of problems;
- incremental processes can be very slow to adapt to environmental change.

## Population-based needs assessment

Figure 7.2 gives a schematic view of the logic of population-based needs assessment. In such broad terms, the theory is simple enough: that the levels of care provided should depend on the characteristics of the population, and that the

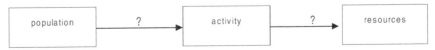

**Figure 7.2** Population-based needs assessment

levels of resources needed will depend on the target levels of provision. The difficult part is to bridge the gaps – the question marks in the diagram.

## Norms for resources

The traditional and most basic approach has been to identify some population-based *norm* or *standard*, and apply it to the local population to determine what the local provision should be. This has generally been done in terms of levels of resources rather than activity. An example of such a standard might be: *25 orthopaedic beds per 100 000 population*.

The main advantage of this approach is that only the most basic data are required: the population size. However, the value of the approach depends very much on where the norms or standards come from. They might be:

- *national averages* – this may be equitable in a narrow sense but may also be inefficient, as the average may be too high or too low to match actual population needs;
- *policy targets* – which may be either below or above the national average; the question then is, what is the justification for the policy?
- *statements of the aspirations* – of particular sectional interest groups (such as orthopaedic surgeons);
- *expert or science-based* – derived from the literature on epidemiology and clinical effectiveness; but this may leave little room for responsiveness to local variations in priorities and patients' attitudes, and to the availability of alternative forms of care and community support.

Another serious disadvantage of simple norms is that the size of a population is by no means the only determinant of its capacity to benefit from health care. Different populations experience different levels of sickness. *Targeted or stratified standards* based on specific groups represent one step forward in this respect. Age is a good predictor of prevalence for most conditions and age-specific standards are quite common. For example: *150 orthopaedic beds per 100 000 population aged 65 and above*. (This does not imply that orthopaedic beds are only required for people aged 65 and above – just that the total number aged 65 and above is a better indicator of population need for orthopaedic surgery than the total number.)

A third disadvantage is that even if resources are provided in line with the norms, this does not imply horizontal equity (equal access for equal need). Providers will vary in the efficiency with which they convert their resources into services.

## Activity 7.2

On your CD there is an Excel file called 'Ch7PopNeed'. In this, the worksheet called 'Population' gives the 1997 population estimates for a whole country and for:

- local area A, an area with a relatively young population including a large new town;
- local area B, a coastal area with a high proportion of more elderly people.

It also gives a five-year projection for local area A. The following figures are given for men and women separately:

- total numbers;
- numbers aged 65 and above;
- a more detailed age breakdown.

Another worksheet called 'Resource norm' shows, in column M, the numbers of orthopaedic beds required in the country as a whole (Figure 7.3). This is derived from the population figures in column D and the norms in column I. The worksheet provides both an all-age norm, and targeted or age-specific norms which separate those aged less than 65 from those aged 65 and above. (These norms are based on national averages, derived from national statistics, but they could just as well be based on policy targets. The calculations involved are the same.)

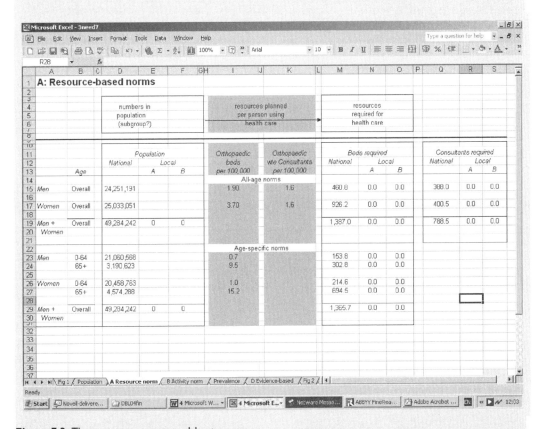

**Figure 7.3** The resource norm spreadsheet

This worksheet also shows, in column Q, the number of consultants required, using a norm based on the average for country, shown in column K. Note that there are no age-specific norms for this.

Use the 'Resource norm' worksheet and the data from the 'Population' worksheet to calculate the number of orthopaedic beds required by local area A implied by:

- the all-age norm
- the age-specific norms.

Do the same for local area B, and compare your answers.

## Feedback

One quick way of doing this is to take the relevant figures from the 'Population' worksheet and copy them by value into the 'Resource norm' spreadsheet, e.g. copy Population!F6 into Resource norm!E15, and Population!F19 into Resource norm!E17, etc. Using the untargeted norms, area B should have around 21 beds to area A's 19, as it has a slightly larger population. But taking age into account changes the picture considerably, with requirements for around 26 beds in area B and 16 in area A. In practice, taking population structure into account will generally have a less marked effect than this.

The norm for consultant specialists in orthopaedics is again based on a national average, dividing the number of whole-time-equivalent (wte) consultants by the size of the national population. In this case it was not possible to derive age-specific averages, as consultants' time is not generally accounted for in terms of patient characteristics. Targeted staffing norms would have to be based on judgements.

### Norms for activity

Now look at the worksheet called 'Activity norm' in Ch7PopNeed. This is an example of the use of national average rates of hip replacement operations, given in column H, to estimate the requirement for a given area. Bradshaw (1972) called this *comparative* or relative needs assessment. The idea is to compare levels of service in your population with levels of service elsewhere.

## Activity 7.3

Once you have an estimate of the requirement for numbers of operations (columns J and K) it is possible to combine these with figures for length of stay and turnover interval to estimate the number of hospital beds in an area that will, on average, be occupied by hip replacement patients (columns Q and R).

1  How many hip replacement operations would you expect in the population of local area A? (Note that you do not need the population data on numbers aged 0–34.)
2  How many beds would you expect to require for hip replacement patients in local area A now, assuming the figures for length of stay and turnover interval given in column N of the Activity norm worksheet?
3  How many beds would you expect to require for hip replacement patients in local area A in five years' time if the age-specific prevalence of the condition, the mean lengths of stay and the turnover intervals all remain about the same?

4 What would happen if in five years' time the mean length of stay has gone down by three days in those aged less than 75? (You can examine this by typing a number of days in the 'change' column – column O – for each age band affected. A positive number of days represents a decrease.)

5 What do you think are the advantages and disadvantages of this approach to needs assessment?

## Feedback

1 You would expect local area A to have about 380 hip replacements. But remember that you have only taken age and gender into account here. There may be other factors to do with, perhaps, ethnicity or levels of physical activity in the population, that have not been 'adjusted for'.

2 The expected requirement for provision in local area A would be around 17 beds.

3 In five years' time the expected requirement would have increased to around 19 beds.

4 The expected requirement would go down to just below 17 beds.

5 The advantages of this approach are:

- It provides a check on horizontal equity: equal access for equal needs.
- It is conceptually simple and can be done on a spreadsheet.
- It only needs data on activity rates from one standard population. So, for example, it can be used to check the equity within a population by applying the population rate to age structures of different subpopulations: different geographic areas, socio-economic or ethnic groups.
- It is possible to consider the effects on the levels of resources required of changes in utilization and changes in medical technology explicitly and separately. For example, in other areas of surgery the requirement for hospital beds has been reduced strikingly by innovations such as reducing lengths of stay, laparoscopic procedures and day surgery.
- For some conditions, current activity rates are appropriate because virtually everyone with the condition receives care. Examples from high income countries are end-stage renal failure (ESRF) and appendicitis. If so, the method can be useful for estimating the effect of possible future changes in the population structure or in the resources needed to provide the service, as you have done here. For example, people with ESRF are surviving longer. What will be the impact of this extended survival on numbers needing dialysis?

The disadvantages of this approach are:

- It is difficult to handle more than three or four explanatory or predictor variables. Also, age and sex may be poor predictors of the variable to be estimated. (Another approach is to estimate using regression equations. This allows many predictor variables, but requires data on many populations.)
- For procedures like elective surgery, it cannot be assumed that current levels of activity are appropriate.

### Epidemiology and norms for 'coverage'

Behind the use of activity-based norms there is a large conceptual leap from population numbers to appropriate levels of health care utilization. You may well have epidemiological data determinants of a disease in a population but not on the determinants of indications for treatment. In this situation there will be a case for using the epidemiological data to make estimates of prevalence, and then make assumptions about the proportion of prevalent cases who will have the indications for treatment. This has been called epidemiologically-based needs assessment, although this phrase has been used by different people in different ways.

### Activity 7.4

Make a copy of the 'Activity norm' worksheet. (Right-click on the sheet's name-tag at the bottom of the screen; click on 'move or copy'; tick the 'create a copy' box, in the 'Before sheet' click on 'D Evidence-based'; and finally click on 'OK'.) Now change the name of the new worksheet from 'B Activity norm (2)' to 'C Coverage norm' (right-click on the name-tag, click on 'rename', move cursor to name tag, click and edit).

Insert five new columns between the population columns (D, E and F) and the utilization column (H), i.e. after column F. The first of these new columns is a spacer, the second for data on age/sex-specific prevalence rates, the third another spacer, the fourth for the actual numbers in the diagnostic group nationally, and the fifth for the 'expected' numbers in your local area, to be calculated from local population * national prevalence. Type in some column headings, and reduce the width of the spacer columns.

Copy the age-specific prevalence rates per 1000 into the new column H (from the spreadsheet called 'Prevalence', ignoring the columns on CIs), and put in some formulae so that new columns J and K give numbers of cases nationally and for local area A.

New column M now becomes 'planned coverage' (i.e. the percentage of people with relevant disease that it is planned to treat this year). Change the heading, and put some rates in the body of the column. You will have to make these rates up to start with, but they should not be more than 100 per cent! Alter the formulae in new columns O and P to give you the numbers planned to receive health care, assuming the planned coverage rates. Now do the following:

1   Compare the numbers in columns O and P to those you had in the 'Activity norm' spreadsheet. What coverage rates would you need in your new spreadsheet to bring the two figures into line with each other? (You will have to use trial and error with the percentages in column M here until the figures in column O and P are about the same as those in the 'Activity Norm' spreadsheet.)
2   What do you think are the strengths and weaknesses of this approach?

**Feedback**

1 This is mainly a question of following the instructions to create a new spreadsheet. You will notice that the coverage rates implied by current levels of activity:

- are broadly similar for men and women;
- seem very low in younger people – of the order of 3 per cent in people aged < 55. This may be because their hip pain is not severe enough for surgery, or because the operation was for some reason other than osteoarthrosis.
- are higher in people aged 65–75 and then drop away sharply in people aged 85 or more. Many people aged 85 or more may be regarded as too fragile for major surgery – or they may have already had replacement operations.

2 The advantages of this approach are:

- For some diseases good epidemiological data are available and almost all prevalent cases will require treatment. If so, this can be a useful approach.
- It is possible to consider the effects of changes in disease prevalence and changes in medical technology explicitly and separately.

The disadvantage of this approach is that for some conditions the relationship between prevalence of disease and need for care is unexpectedly weak. In one of the first needs assessment studies, Willcock (1979) examined the link between cases of osteoarthrosis (OA) of the hip and need for hip replacement. He carried out a survey of records in primary care and found that of 46 prevalent cases of hip OA, 22 of them were below the severity threshold for surgery, 11 were unfit for surgery, four had already had surgery, and five were ineligible on other grounds. Of the remaining four, two were on the waiting list. (One didn't want surgery, leaving only one 'iceberg' case of unrecognized need for care.)

### Indications for treatment and coverage

The following extracts are from a paper by Frankel and colleagues (1999).

 **Need for and provision of total hip replacement in England**

*Introduction*

Total hip replacement is one of the commonest elective surgical procedures; around 43,500 primary operations are done each year in English NHS and independent hospitals. There are some concerns about effectiveness, particularly with respect to prostheses that have not been fully evaluated and to the proper indications for treatment, but this procedure is generally regarded as unquestionably cost-effective.

Potential demand can be estimated from data on use of health services, but this is clearly a circular process. Epidemiological studies of the distribution of radiological osteoarthritis of the hip have shown that prevalence increases with age, with 5 per cent or more of the population older than 65 years showing evidence of severe change on radiography. Population requirements for surgery cannot be estimated from such findings, since the relation between radiographic change, symptoms, and function is uncertain.

*Methods*

Two separate published sets of criteria for total hip replacement surgery have been used: the criteria agreed in 1995 at the US National Institutes of Health consensus conference (NIH method); and the New Zealand priority criteria for major joint replacement surgery (New Zealand score). To estimate population requirements for surgery, the measured prevalence of symptoms and functional limitation in the population were related to these published criteria. The NIH consensus conference aimed to find out the current indications for total hip replacement. The conclusion of the 13-member panel, 27 experts, and conference audience of 425 was that candidates for elective total hip replacement should have moderate to severe persistent pain, disability, or both, not substantially relieved by an extended course of non-surgical (medical) management.

The New Zealand score has a maximum value of 100; higher scores reflect more severe disease. Cut-off points of 43 and 55 were selected before analysis to reflect moderate and severe disease, respectively (to date, no cut-off point for access to surgery has been agreed in New Zealand). Illustrative examples of the degrees of pain and disability that may be expected with such scores are shown in Table 7.1. The number potentially requiring surgery was then modified to exclude those who were unfit for surgery (reported chest tightness, wheeze, breathlessness, chest pain, or palpitations many times a day or all the time); those who had not had an adequate trial of medical therapy; and those who had said they would not accept surgical intervention if it were offered.

**Table 7.1** Degrees of pain and disability associated with New Zealand scores of 55 and 43

| Characteristic | Max score | Cut-off at score 55 | | Cut-off at score 43 | |
| --- | --- | --- | --- | --- | --- |
| | | Description | Points | Description | Points |
| Degree of pain | 20 | Moderate to severe | 14 | Moderate | 9 |
| Occurrence of pain | 20 | Regular at night | 20 | Regular at night | 20 |
| Walking ability | 10 | Can walk for 11–30 m | 4 | Can walk for 11–30 m | 4 |
| Functional limitations (e.g. managing stairs, sitting to standing, recreation/hobbies) | 10 | Moderate limitations | 4 | Mild limitations | 2 |
| Pain on examination | 10 | Mild | 2 | Mild | 2 |
| Other problems, e.g. reduced range of movement, deformity, limp | 10 | Moderate | 5 | Mild | 2 |
| Other joints involved | 10 | None | 0 | None | 0 |
| Ability to work, give care to dependants, live independently: difficulty | 10 | Threatened but not immediately | 6 | Not threatened but more difficult | 4 |
| Total | 100 | | 55 | | 43 |

Source: Frankel et al. (1999).

*Results*

Table 7.2 shows the population prevalence and estimated annual incidence of hip disease that may be amenable to primary total hip replacement. These rates were derived according to the NIH method and the two cut-off points for the New Zealand score, with the assumption that non-attenders and attenders are alike. Right-sided disease was more common than left-sided disease, as has been found elsewhere.

**Table 7.2** Population prevalence of severe hip disease per 1000 people

| | Rate per 1000 (95% CI) | | |
| --- | --- | --- | --- |
| | New Zealand score >55 | New Zealand score >43 | NIH method |
| Prevalence right hip | | | |
| Men | 7.6 (4.9–10.3) | 13.7 (10.2–17.3) | 5.9 (3.5–8.2) |
| Women | 12.6 (9.4–15.8) | 25.8 (21.2–30.4) | 12.6 (9.4–15.8) |
| All | 10.1 (8.0–12.2) | 20.4 (17.4–23.3) | 9.5 (7.4–11.5) |
| Prevalence right hip | | | |
| Men | 7.6 (4.9–10.3) | 11.3 (8.1–14.6) | 6.6 (4.1–9.1) |
| Women | 9.2 (6.4–11.9) | 22.4 (18.2–26.7) | 8.7 (6.0–11.4) |
| All | 8.5 (6.6–10.4) | 17.0 (14.3–19.7) | 7.8 (5.9–9.7) |
| Prevalence right hip | | | |
| Men | 11.9 (8.6–15.2) | 19.5 (15.2–23.7) | 9.7 (6.7–12.7) |
| Women | 18.1 (14.2–21.9) | 37.2 (31.7–42.7) | 17.0 (13.2–20.7) |
| All | 15.2 (12.7–17.8) | 29.0 (25.4–32.5) | 13.6 (11.2–16.1) |

Source: Frankel et al. (1999).

In 1994–95 there were 32,500 procedures for primary total hip replacement in the English NHS. An additional 11,000 procedures a year are carried out in the independent sector, resulting in a total of 43,500 procedures per year currently carried out in England.

*Discussion*

Total hip replacement is one of the most effective and most desired surgical interventions ... This study reports estimated requirements for primary total hip replacement from a large population-based probability sample; the study combined self-reported morbidity with clinical examination and incidence estimates. The crude estimates of incident indications for total hip replacement exceeded current operation rates in England by between 12 per cent and 49 per cent depending on the criteria applied (Table 7.3). However, when these rates were adjusted to take account of other influences on the decision to recommend surgery (fitness for surgery, completion of a trial of medication, and the person's own willingness to undergo surgery), the estimates of incident cases ranged from 3 per cent to 11 per cent in excess of current operation rates. Our preferred reflection of surgical practice is a New Zealand score of 55 or more; with this criterion the required surgical activity exceeds current activity by about 6 per cent, when the above three influences are taken into account ...

This study suggests that there is no fundamental reason why primary total hip replacement surgery should be denied to those who would benefit from it, provided that there is agreement on the indications consistent with the most effective treatment. The rationing debate could usefully shift from the current preoccupation with mechanisms for implementing the denial of treatment and towards demanding explicit justification of any long-term rationing in particular areas of effective care.

**Table 7.3** Estimate* of annual incident hip disease requiring primary total hip replacement surgery in the population of England aged 35 to 85

| | Annual incident cases of hip disease (95% CI)* | | |
| --- | --- | --- | --- |
| | New Zealand score >55 | New Zealand score >43 | NIH method |
| Estimated population incidence | 54.0 (35.9–72.1) | 64.8 (44.6–85.0) | 48.8 (30.9–66.6) |
| Positive preference for surgery only | 49.4 (30.2–68.5) | 54.3 (33.9–74.8) | 46.2 (27.2–65.2) |
| Fit for surgery | 52.4 (32.9–71.8) | 60.4 (38.9–81.8) | 48.6 (29.2–68.0) |
| On medication in previous year | 51.1 (31.7–70.5) | 56.7 (35.9–77.6) | 46.8 (27.7–65.9) |
| Positive preference and fit | 47.9 (29.0–66.8) | 51.3 (31.2–71.4) | 45.6 (26.7–64.5) |
| Positive preference and medication | 47.3 (28.5–66.2) | 49.9 (30.2–69.7) | 45.0 (26.2–63.7) |
| Fit on medication | 49.2 (30.2–68.3) | 54.1 (33.7–74.6) | 46.1 (27.1–65.0) |
| Positive preference, fit and on medication. | 46.2 (27.5–64.9) | 48.5 (28.9–68.0) | 44.6 (25.9–63.2) |

Note:* Expressed as 1000s of joints. Estimated from prevalent cases by the New Zealand and NIH methods, with allowance for patients' preferences for surgery, patients' fitness for surgery, and patients who would be amenable to medical therapy.

Source: Frankel et al. (1999).

Now look at the spreadsheet called 'Evidence-based'. This is an attempt to estimate the likely requirement for hip replacement in local area A, based on a combination of the findings of the paper by Frankel and colleagues and some speculative assumptions about how age groups differ in terms of their desire for surgery. You can see that in this model there are far more intermediate stages than in the others. This is because more of the various factors and assumptions underpinning any needs assessment are made explicit.

## Activity 7.5

Use the model to answer the following:

1 How many people in the population of local area A would you estimate both want hip replacement and have the indications for it? How does this compare with the 'expected' figure for hip replacement operations from the worksheet called 'Activity norm'? What do you infer from this?

2 What data are used and what are the sources of error involved in the derived estimates?

3 Where do the judgements come into this evidence-based approach to needs assessment?

4 What do you think are the problems with this approach?

## ↻ Feedback

1 About 595. This is a lot higher than the figure of 380 that you estimated in Activity 2 by applying the national average rates. If the indications for surgery (or treatment thresholds) used are accepted, it would seem as though the English health service is some way below providing hip replacements for all those that could benefit from it. However, these national averages are only for operations carried out in the public sector. As Frankel and colleagues point out, large numbers of hip replacements are also carried out in private hospitals. This is partly because at the time people often had to wait a long time for elective surgery in the public sector. (If you include the operations done in private hospitals, the figure of 595 may be quite a good match to the number actually done.) Thus, implicit in the level of provision is a view of what proportion of the population's need for this procedure the provider in question should cater for. In this worksheet this is expressed as % 'coverage' (in column AB). Judgements about coverage tend to be implicit, but are revealed by this kind of analysis.

2 This approach brings in data on the *prevalence of the indications* for surgery and also on attitudes to surgery: whether those with the necessary indications actually want surgery or not. These data are based on a sample of 40 general practices which, although large, may be biased. There is no information on how the practices involved were recruited; maybe their patients were atypical. It is also subject to substantial sampling error, with quite wide 95 per cent confidence intervals shown in Table 7.3. Also, here again, the only characteristics of the local populations that are taken into account are age and gender. You do not know how much of the variation in prevalence between areas can be explained by these two variables alone.

3 This approach involves judgements about the *indications for surgery* and the *level of coverage by the health care system*. Frankel et al. (1999) found that for hip replacement the number of operations required was reasonably robust to choice of treatment threshold, but this is not always the case. Sanderson et al. (1997) report on a needs assessment for prostatectomy, a major operation to reduce urinary symptoms in middle-aged and older men. The indications for this operation are largely based on severity of symptoms and flow measurements. An American consensus panel suggested that a score of 8 or more on a 7-question symptom questionnaire (the AUA7) indicated that surgery should be discussed with the patient. An English panel suggested a threshold symptom score of 11, and the eligibility criterion in the only published randomized trial was a score of 15. Urinary symptoms are very common but some men find them more bothersome than others, even when they are severe. Table 7.4 shows

**Table 7.4** Results: 'need' for prostatectomy in a population of 250,000

| | Prevalence | | | Incidence | |
|---|---|---|---|---|---|
| | AUA7 8+ | 11+ | 15+ | 11+ | 15+ |
| symptoms of BPH | 11,500 | 7600 | 4000 | | |
| symptoms, at least small bother | | 3800 | 3000 | | |
| symptoms, at least medium bother | | 1800 | 1750 | 640 | |
| symptoms, at least medium bother and probably/definitely wants surgery | | 630 | 610 | 350 | 200 |

Source: Sanderson et al. (1997).

how the estimated numbers of prevalent cases in a population varied widely with changes in the threshold symptom score and in how bothersome the men find their symptoms, but also with whether or not the men would 'definitely or probably' want the operation if offered it. This is an effective procedure, but it is a major one with a significant risk of causing impotence, and urinary symptoms of this kind quite commonly go into spontaneous remission.

4 In terms of problems with the evidence-based approach, it is very demanding of information. It requires:

(a) *clear and accepted indications for treatment.* The problem is that doctors often do not agree about indications. There is not enough research on subgroups and outcomes and many do not accept what research results there are. Also indications for treatment should depend on expected outcomes and, in general, there will be very limited data on the outcomes of any particular hospital or doctor. The assumption has to be made that local services produce results similar to pooled research data or in line with expert consensus.

(b) *the local prevalence of people with these indications and information on who wants the treatment in question.* Such local data as may be available usually relate to levels of health care activity or disease, not indications for or acceptability of a procedure. They may be subject to sampling error and bias. And while some conditions – such as fractures – are either present or not, many others, such as hypertension and diabetes, are defined by threshold values. Someone whose measurement is above this threshold value has the disease, and below it they don't. In some cases the indication for treatment is severity of symptoms, defined as having a symptom score above a given level. In these situations the estimated numbers in a population needing health care can be highly sensitive to the choice of defining threshold. Furthermore, acceptability to the patient may depend on how the intervention is described.

 **Activity 7.6**

Both Frankel et al. and Sanderson et al. limited themselves to estimating the numbers of people in their populations who needed a particular procedure. However, this is not a sufficient basis for decisions about what level of services to provide. What additional information is necessary for this?

 **Feedback**

Strategic decision makers have to determine the priority to be given to hip replacement in the context of the overall provision of health care to the population; they have to consider vertical equity as well as horizontal. To do this properly they would also need to know:

• the nature and extent of benefits that can be expected;

- the relative values attached to the benefits from hip replacement (less pain, more mobility) compared to benefits from other kinds of intervention;
- the costs of providing care for this number of cases.

The first of these should be available from the health services research literature, although as you have seen, strictly it is the quality of the local outcomes that are relevant here. There may be information on relative values from QALY or DALY exercises for example, but, again, these may not be the same as local values. There may be information on costs from the local information systems or industry tariffs.

You can see why these difficult questions, about how the balance of local health care provision should be tilted one way or another, involve large measures of judgement. The question then is whether there are 'good' ways of arriving at these judgements. Consensus development, and the problem structuring methods of the kind described in Chapter 3 may have roles to play in this.

## Summary

In this chapter you have learned how strategic planning and intervention are required to ensure that health services are efficient and equitable. You have seen how the assessment of health needs can assist in the planning of health care delivery, and how corporate needs assessment attempts to balance the interests and pressures of all interested parties. You have also learned about population-based approaches and how models of increasing complexity can be built so as to base assessment on epidemiological data, on indications for care, and on the acceptability of particular procedures. Figure 7.4 (overleaf) provides an overview of these.

All population-based methods involve some element of value judgement and these are indicated in italics in Figure 7.4. Evidence-based needs assessment makes less sweeping assumptions than other methods and is the most appealing in theory but is very demanding of data and vulnerable to choices about indications, particularly if threshold values are involved.

The modelling involved in population-based assessment is technically straight-forward but corporate needs assessment is still the predominant approach. This is partly because there are so few data on which to base a rigorous population-based approach and partly because the processes and structures required to produce the necessary judgements about indications, coverage, etc. are underdeveloped.

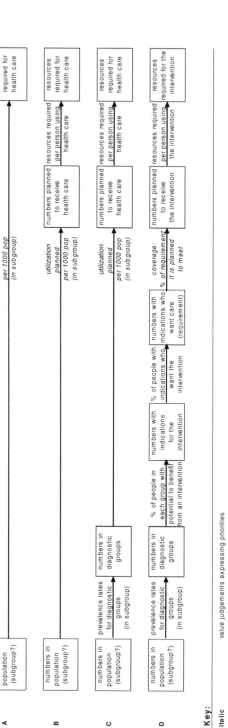

**Figure 7.4** Different approaches to estimating resources required to meet population needs

**Key:**

Italic:    value judgements expressing priorities

Boxed:    local figures, established by local studies, or estimated using data from studies elsewhere

Unboxed:    data from surveys or ??nomic studies used for estimating local figures

*    subgroups chosen to be predictive of incidence/prevalence, to allow local estimation from surveys elsewhere, eg age group

A:    Resource-related policies (norms)    the amount of resources provided follows from the decision as to resources per 1000 population
eg: 1 orthopaedic bed per 1,000 population (or with subgroups: 1 bed/20,000 aged < 75, and 1 bed/1000 aged 75+

B:    Activity/utilisation-related    The amount of resources provided follows from the decision on utilisation per 1000 population,
eg: 20 hip replacements per year per 1000 population aged over 75.

C:    Disease-related policies (epidemiological)    the amount of resources provided follows from the decision as to the % of those with a given condition to be provided for
eg: 200 hip replacements per year per 1000 people with (severe?) OA of the hip.

D:    Needs-related policies (evidence-based)    the amount of resources provided follows from the decision as to the % of those who could benefit from care
that should be treated in any one year.

# References

Bradshaw J (1972) A taxonomy of social need, in McLachlan G (ed.) *Problems and Progress in Medical Care*, 7th series. Oxford: Oxford University Press.

Culyer A (1976) *Need and the National Health Service: Economics and social choice*, pp. 11–12. Oxford: Martin Robinson.

Frankel S, Eachus J, Pearson J et al. (1999) Population requirement for primary hip-replacement surgery: a cross-sectional study. *Lancet* 353: 1304–9.

Matthew GK (1971) Measuring need and evaluating services, in McLachlan G (ed.) *Problems and Progress in Medical Care*, 6th series. Oxford: Oxford University Press.

Sanderson CFB, Hunter DJW, McKee CM and Black NA (1997) Limitations of epidemiological needs assessment: the case of prostatectomy. *Medical Care* 35: 669–85.

Whitehead M (1992) The concepts and principles of equity and health. *International Journal of Health Services* 22: 429–45.

Willcock GK (1979) The prevalence of osteoarthrosis of the hip requiring total hip replacement. *International Journal of Epidemiology* 8: 247–50.

# 8 | Balanced service provision

## Overview

In Chapter 4 you learned about ways of choosing one option from many. In Chapter 7 you learned about ways of determining the appropriate levels of resource or activity for a particular service, the implicit assumption being that the necessary resources could be found, at least in the medium term. However, where there are limits to the availability of resources, doing more of one thing will generally mean doing less of another. In this chapter you will consider the question of how to achieve the best mix or balance of service provision when resources are limited. Decision makers may have to address questions such as: given the resources available, the health needs or demands of the population served, and the scope for altering the balance of provision, *which* services should be provided? *How much* of each type of service should be provided? Where do the resource bottlenecks arise? And what will be gained by relieving a given bottleneck?

## Learning objectives

**By the end of this chapter, you will be better able to:**

- **explain the circumstances in which 'best mix' problems arise in health care**
- **describe the linear programming formulation of this type of problem**
- **assess the strengths and weaknesses of one type of model designed to support health care planning decisions**

## Key terms

**Constraints** Upper or lower limits on the level of a particular activity.

**Feasible region** All the possible combinations of values of a variable that are consistent with a given set of constraints.

**Linear programming** An approach to finding feasible and, in particular, the best solutions when the constraints and objective function are linear.

**Objective function** A mathematical function of the values of a variable which represents an objective to be either maximized (e.g. health gain) or minimized (e.g. cost).

## Best mix or balance in the provision of health care

Health care involves the use of many different kinds of resources in different ways and in different settings, for different types of patient. For example, non-specialist doctors-in-training, nurses and domestic staff take on different roles in looking after patients. Some tasks currently done by nurses might be done by domestic staff; others might be done by doctors; and vice versa. Some patients looked after in hospital could be cared for in the community and vice versa; each type of patient involves different amounts of doctor, nursing and domestic time, and derives different benefits from the care that they receive. Some patients not receiving care at all could benefit from it, and so on.

In this situation, questions arise such as:

- What is the best mix of services to provide, given current levels of resources? (for example, should you do 40 per cent as hospital care and 60 per cent as community care? Or should you alter this balance?)
- If you wanted to treat 20 per cent more of patients of type X, what extra resources would be needed?
- If you employed Y more nurses, how many more patients of type X could you treat and what resources would be freed up for use elsewhere?

Answering these kinds of question can become very complicated if there are many resources and many alternative uses for them and many *constraints*: limits on the amount of particular resources that can be used. Management scientists have devised ways of setting up such problems as systems of equations and solving them. Of course, health services are not industrial plant, with well-understood and tightly controlled production processes. Even if more were known about the production functions involved, they would be naturally 'fuzzy' and elastic, so that the validity of describing a hospital's 'production' as equations that can be solved mathematically is debateable.

Nonetheless, there are some situations in which this way of thinking about the problem can be helpful. You will start by considering a simplified example and then read about an application of the approach in reality.

Consider an operation that can be done either as day surgery or as an in-patient procedure. For some of the more severely ill or fragile patients, day surgery may be inappropriate, while some of the fitter patients may have a strong preference for day surgery; but in many cases there will be a proportion of patients who could be treated either way.

The day procedure may be less demanding of hospital resources but often it will be more demanding of community resources. Resources are not unlimited, however. Thus, although there may be different kinds of reason for wanting to increase the proportion of day surgery cases (e.g. patient preference, cost saving, avoidance of infection), there may be limited scope for this if there are, for example, insufficient community nurses.

To simplify, assume that each procedure has equally good outcomes. In this case the sorts of question that can arise are:

- How many of these procedures could be done as day cases, given current levels of resources?

- If you wanted to do 20 per cent more procedures as day cases, what additional resources would be needed in the community, and what resources would be freed up in hospital?

 **Activity 8.1**

Surgery for varicose veins is one such procedure. Table 8.1 shows the different kinds of staff involved and provides estimates of the amounts of their time that each case involves, for day surgery in the first column and for in-patient surgery in the second. It also shows, in the right-hand column, estimates of the maximum amounts of time available for this procedure in a particular hospital for each category of staff. Looking at Table 8.1, work out the maximum number of varicose vein operations that can be done per week in this hospital. (Don't spend more than a few minutes on this.)

**Table 8.1** Types of resources involved in providing surgery for varicose veins

|  | Day care Hours per patient | In-patient Hours per patient | Constraints Hours available per week |
|---|---|---|---|
| Specialists | 0 | 0.5 | 5 |
| Junior doctors | 2 | 2.5 | 30 |
| Hospital nurses | 4 | 8 | 80 |
| Theatre | 1 | 1 | 20 |
| Community nurses | 10 | 0 | 100 |
| Ambulances | 1 | 0 | 12 |

 **Feedback**

The answer is 14. If you worked this out, you did well! But this is a relatively simple problem with only two options (day versus in-patient surgery) and six types of resources. Bigger problems need a methodical approach.

## Formulating the problem in terms of linear constraints

Suppose that you were to schedule $x_1$ cases per week to be done as day surgery and $x_2$ to be done as in-patients. You know that *specialist surgeons* take 0.5 hours for each in-patient case and are unwilling to spend more than five hours per week on this procedure. The implication is that no more than $5/0.5 = 10$ in-patient varicose vein operations can be done per week, so $x_2 \leqslant 10$. For *hospital nurses*, each day case takes four hours and each in-patient eight hours, so the total time they would spend on varicose vein patients per week would be $4x_1 + 8x_2$, and this must be $\leqslant 80$ hours. The complete set of equations, or more correctly, inequalities, is set out in Table 8.2.

**Table 8.2** Resource and constraints in equation/inequality form

|  | Day care | | In-patient | | Constraints |
|---|---|---|---|---|---|
| Specialists | 0 | $x_1$ + | 0.5 | $x_2$  <= | 5 |
| Junior doctors | 2 | $x_1$ + | 2.5 | $x_2$  <= | 30 |
| Hospital nurses | 4 | $x_1$ + | 8 | $x_2$  <= | 80 |
| Theatre | 1 | $x_1$ + | 1 | $x_2$  <= | 20 |
| Community nurses | 10 | $x_1$ + | 0 | $x_2$  <= | 100 |
| Ambulances | 1 | $x_1$ + | 0 | $x_2$  <= | 12 |

With only the two activities, day surgery and in-patient surgery for varicose veins, you can use a diagram to represent the problem. In Figure 8.1, the numbers of day cases are on the vertical axis and the number of in-patient cases on the horizontal axis. Each point on the graph represents some particular 'balance of production'; the point (4, 8) would represent four in-patient cases and eight day cases per week.

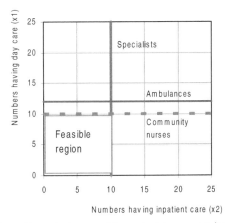

**Figure 8.1** Mix of day and in-patient care, with constraints on specialists, ambulances and community nurses

Each line in the diagram represents a constraint. You know that you cannot do more than 10 in-patient procedures per week or you will run out of specialist surgeon time. Thus the vertical line rising from the value 10 on the $x_2$ axis represents the *specialist surgeon constraint*. You cannot plan to produce anywhere on the diagram to the right of this line.

Likewise, you cannot plan to produce anywhere on the diagram above the line marked 'ambulances' that runs horizontally from the value 12 on the $x_1$ axis because day cases take on average one hour of ambulance time and, from Table 8.2, you only have up to 12 hours per week available for this.

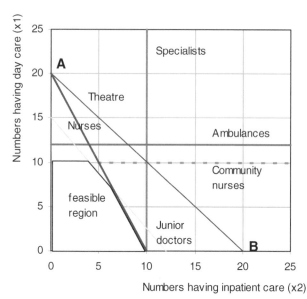

**Figure 8.2** Mix of day and in-patient care, with additional constraints on hospital resources

Figure 8.2 shows three more constraints. They are still represented by straight lines but because they involve combinations of day and in-patient surgery the lines are sloped. To see why, consider the operating theatre constraint. You cannot do more than 20 varicose vein operations per week. You could do one of the following combinations:

- 0 in-patients and 20 day cases (the point (0,20) at A on the $x_1$ axis);
- 1 day case and 19 in-patients (the point (1,19));
- 10 day cases and 10 in-patient (the point (10,10));
- 20 day cases and 0 in-patients (the point (20,0) at B on the $x_2$ axis).

If you plot all these points, they lie on the line AB. You can draw similar lines for:

- hospital nurses (from (10,0) to (0,20)) because 80/8 = 10 and 80/4 = 20;
- junior doctors (from (12,0) to (0,15)).

These lines are all maximum constraints – you cannot go above or outside any of them. If you take them all together, you find that they define an area at the bottom left-hand corner of the diagram which contains all the combinations of in-patient and day case surgery rates that are possible, given the set of constraints. This area, which has been shaded, is called the *feasible region*. As long as you are within this, you have not violated any of the constraints.

Now try using Figure 8.2 to answer some questions.

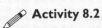

## Activity 8.2

What is the maximum number of varicose vein operations that can be carried out within existing resource limits? How many day cases and how many in-patients will this include?

## Feedback

The answer is 14, consisting of 10 day cases and 4 in-patients. For $x_1$ day cases per week and $x_2$ in-patients, the total number of varicose vein operations per week $= x_1 + x_2$.

Now look at Figure 8.3. A number of sloping parallel lines have been drawn. These are the lines that join sets of values of $x_1$ and $x_2$ for which

$$x_1 + x_2 = n$$

where n = 12 for the inner line, 14 for the next one, 16 for the next and 18 for the outermost.

These lines represent the possible ways of carrying out 12, 14, 16 and 18 varicose vein operations respectively. Notice how the line for n = 12 passes through the feasible

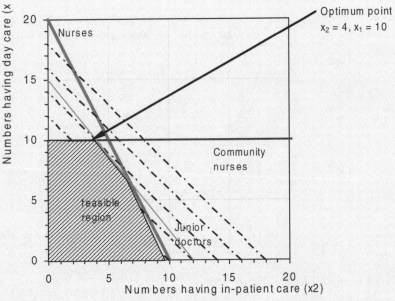

**Figure 8.3** Mix of day and in-patient care, showing lines of constant surgical activity

region. In general this means there is more than one way of carrying out 12 operations within the constraints. The line for n = 16 lies entirely beyond the feasible region, so there is no way of carrying out 16 operations. However, the line for n = 14 just touches the feasible region, at the point (4,10). This means that it is possible to carry out 14 operations but only by doing 4 in-patient operations and 10 day cases. This point (4,10) is indicated as the optimum because it represents the only way of doing 14 operations without violating any constraints.

 **Activity 8.3**

Suppose you wanted to do 16 vein operations per week. What additional resources would be needed?

 **Feedback**

You need to extend the feasible region so that the line for n = 16 goes through or touches it. You can see from Figure 8.3 that first constraints to 'relax' are junior doctors and community nurses, because it is at the intersection of these two con-straints that the optimum point lies. (You are inside the constraint lines for the other resources, which implies that you are working at below capacity in these respects; the constraints involved are redundant.)

To do 16 vein operations per week, you need 5 hours more junior doctor time and 20 hours more community nurse time. This position is shown in Figure 8.4, with the

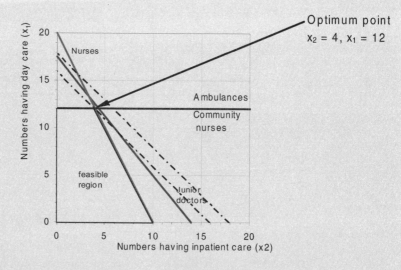

----------- Lines of constant surgical activity

**Figure 8.4** Mix of day and in-patient care with increased resource levels

constraint lines for these two resources moved to new positions. The community nurse constraint now coincides with the ambulance constraint. The optimum is at (4,12), and with 12 day cases the allowances for ambulances, hospital nurses and community nurses are completely used up, and the allowance for junior doctors is almost used up. Thus, a smaller proportion of the resources allocated to vein operations are unused.

## Activity 8.4

Go back to the resource constraints set out in Table 8.1 and Figure 8.3. Now suppose that the costs of the various components of care are as shown in Table 8.3. You are contracted to provide varicose vein surgery for *12 patients per week*. What is the cheapest way of doing this?

Note that this activity introduces two new elements:

- a new minimum constraint: a new line beyond which the feasible region must lie, as you have to produce at least 12 operations. This is represented by the line $x_1 + x_2 \geq 12$.
- a new objective: try drawing a series of parallel lines of constant cost, similar to the lines of constant numbers of operations shown in Figure 8.3.

**Table 8.3** Costs of the different resources involved

|  | Unit cost | Day care | | In-patient | | Constraints |
|---|---|---|---|---|---|---|
|  | per hour | Hours | Cost per patient | Hours | Cost per patient | Hours available per week |
| Specialists | 40 | 0 | 0 | 0.5 | 20 | 5 |
| Junior doctors | 20 | 2 | 40 | 2.5 | 20 | 30 |
| Hospital nurses | 10 | 4 | 40 | 8 | 10 | 80 |
| Theatre | 180 | 1 | 180 | 1 | 180 | 20 |
| Community nurses | 10 | 10 | 100 | 0 | 10 | 100 |
| Ambulances | 60 | 1 | 60 | 0 | 60 | 12 |
| Indirect costs |  |  | 180 |  | 700 |  |
| Total |  |  | 600 |  | 1 000 |  |

## Feedback

Figure 8.5 shows the new minimum constraint on numbers of operations performed as a dashed line, which provides an inner limit to the shape of the feasible region.

Now if day cases cost £600 and in-patients cost £1000, then the total cost of vein surgery per week is:

$$600x_1 + 1000x_2.$$

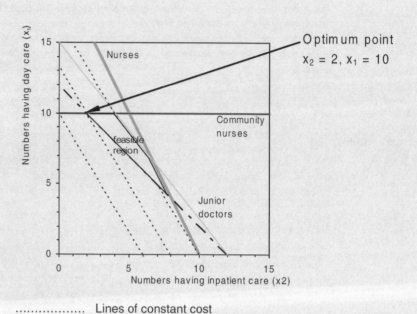

.................. Lines of constant cost

**Figure 8.5** Mix of day and in-patient care, given minimum number of operations

You can thus draw a series of lines of constant cost, of the form:

$$600x_1 + 1000x_2 = C$$

These are shown in Figure 8.5 for C = £6000, £8000 and £10,000, the outer lines representing higher costs.

This time, notice that at the lower value of C, no section of the constant cost line passes through the feasible region. The implication is that you cannot provide the necessary 12 operations for £6000. With C = £8000 the line just touches the feasible region at (2,10), the point indicated as being the optimum. This represents 2 in-patient operations at £1000 each and 10 day cases at £600 each, the minimum total cost subject to the constraints you have been given. In retrospect, this makes sense. It implies doing as much as you can of the cheaper option and then using any resources you have left over on the more expensive one.

Now you want to explore the effect of freeing some of the bottlenecks or relaxing some constraints. Rather than draw more graphs you will do this by using the Excel Solver. This is an Excel Add-in, one of a number of such facilities that allow Excel to do some common forms of data analysis for you.

✎ **Activity 8.5**

Open the file 'Ch8LinProg' on your CD and select the spreadsheet called 'Solver I'. The yellow part of the table provides the data for the problem and the green area is where you want Solver to put the answers. You will notice that three of the constraints have been changed. The upper limit on community nurse time has been raised from 100 to 125 hours per week, the limit of junior doctor hours raised from 30 to 35, and the limit on hospital nurses from 80 to 90. To start with, no patients are being treated.

First, check whether Solver has been installed on your computer. Go to the menu bar at the top of the screen and click on Tools, Solver. This should bring up the Solver Parameters screen. If when you click on Solver you get an error message, or if Solver is not an option on your Tools menu, you need to install it. Click on Tools, Add-Ins. On the Add-Ins interface screen, tick the Solver Add-In box and then OK.

Now, place the cursor over cell F13, check that it contains the formula B13+C13, the total numbers treated. This is what you want to maximize. Open Solver and type F13 into the window for target cell and then specify the control variables in the 'By Changing Cells' window. These are $x_1$ and $x_2$, the numbers of day and inpatient cases, so you type in B13:C13. Now you need the constraints. Column F shows the usage: how much of each resource is used for given values of the control variables. For example F5 = B5*B$13+C5*C$13.

The constraints are thus $F$5 <= $E$5 etc. To add a new constraint:

- Click on Add on the Solver Parameters screen to bring up the Add Constraint form.
- Fill in the 'form' for the first constraint. There is a drop-down menu in the middle of the form which allows you to specify whether the value in the 'cell reference' window should be >=, = or <= the value in the 'constraint' window.
- Click on Add to add another constraint, or on OK to finish and go back to Solver Parameters.

Once you have all your constraints in place, click on Solve. Solver's solution should appear in cells B13 and C13, with the total numbers treated in F13. (In some situations you may find that you have been offered a solution with a negative value of numbers of cases treated. This is an example of how computers can give useless answers unless you tell them how to recognize useless solutions in advance and rule them out. To avoid this particular problem you would need to add two more constraints: $x_1 >= 0$ and $x_2 >= 0$.)

### Feedback

The solution should be 12 day care patients and 4.4 in-patients. However, you cannot treat 0.4 patients. You need to make sure that the solution is in whole numbers (integers).

### Activity 8.6

Do this by adding another constraint: that the control variables, B13:C13, are integers. In the constraints form, put B13:C13 in the cell reference. Then click on the drop-down arrow in the middle field of the form and choose 'int'. 'Integer' will appear in the right-hand field. Now click on Solve.

**Feedback**

The solution that comes up should be 12 day cases and 4 in-patients, a total of 16. The spreadsheet 'Solver 2' in Ch8LinProg produces this. If you had problems setting up your constraints, have a look at the Solver Parameters screen for this spreadsheet. You may have to scroll down to see all the constraints.

**Activity 8.7**

Now go back to the question of how to minimize the cost of carrying out 12 operations a week. Remember that a day case costs £600 and an in-patient case £1000. You need to add these costs to your data and use them to create a new target cell, the total cost of operations performed; you also need to add another constraint to ensure that at least 12 operations are done, and to select the 'min' box instead of the 'max'.

**Feedback**

You can see how this might be done on the spreadsheet 'Solver 3'. The lowest cost solution is, unsurprisingly, to do as many as you can using the cheaper operation. With the resources that you now have, you can do all 12. However, the surgeons may well say that there are always some patients who cannot be treated on a day case basis. It is quite common that a proposed solution makes people realize that there is another constraint that they had forgotten about. After due reflection and/or consultation of records, they argue that at least 3 cases per week have to be done as in-patients. You need to introduce a new constraint, $x_2 >= 3$, and try again. This gives 9 day and 3 in-patient cases.

## Linear programming

The problem you have just considered is a simple example of a more general type that management scientists describe as a *programming* problem. The word programme means a predetermined set of mathematical steps rather than the more general *computer* program. But as it happens in this case it also has something in common with, say, a concert programme – a deliberately chosen, balanced mix of items. The essential ingredients are:

- a set of different types of resources to be used for different jobs;
- at least some of the jobs can be done in more than one way, i.e. by using different packages of resources;
- a set of constraints on availability of at least some resources;
- the powers to switch resources between jobs.

The objective of the decision maker is to use these powers to achieve one or more of the following:

- improve quality of care and/or numbers treated;
- avoid bottlenecks;
- reduce costs.

To do this, the decision maker has to be able to answer questions such as, given the resources available and constraints:

- Which jobs should be done?
- How many of each type of job should be done?
- Where do the resource bottlenecks arise?
- What will be gained by relieving a given bottleneck?

In the varicose veins problem that you have just considered, the constraints were represented by straight lines. This was because there were no returns to scale; the average number of hours that a nurse or doctor spent on each case did not vary with the throughput in the hospital, i.e. with $x_1$ or $x_2$. The *objective functions* (maximize $x_1 + x_2$ to maximize throughput; minimize $600x_1 + 1000x_2$ to minimize costs) could also be represented by straight lines. Thus this was a *linear* programming problem. In theory it is quite easy to find the optimum solution to a problem of this kind, because the optimum will always be where two or more constraints intersect.

As you have seen, in health care there is almost never enough reliable information about *production functions* and *objective functions* for optimal solutions based on linear programming to warrant much credibility. But as an approach to identifying a *feasible region* of possible solutions and of identifying the critical constraints and the effects of relaxing them, the technique can work well.

## The balance of care model

In Activity 8.1 you worked with a simplified and rather unrealistic hypothetical example of how linear programming can illuminate best mix problems. Now you will learn about a real computer-based planning model that was developed by operational researchers at the Department of Health in England during the 1970s. Since then it has been used in Spain, the Netherlands, Italy and Australia. In its longish life it has been through a good deal of development, partly aimed at simplifying its use by building in more data and partly to take advantage of the improved user interfaces and portability offered by more recent software and computers. In its latest form it is used by a firm of specialist health care management consultants in conjunction with a series of local planning workshops.

Cropper and Forte (1997) describe a version of the model that has been developed to support planning of care for elderly people. Others have been developed to support planning for AIDS and HIV, for example, Tramarin et al. 1997.) This is not for planning acute services, but for the kinds of long-term care needed by substantial numbers of elderly people.

The first step in the approach is to identify groups in the elderly population with different care needs. In the model these groups are defined primarily in terms of dependencies:

The number of community nurses per 10,000 people over 65, for example, indicates nothing about whether this resource is appropriately targeted to those who require it – and a large proportion of the population may not have any need at all. What is important is to relate information on services to levels of dependency in the population.

A working definition of dependency can be taken on two principal dimensions: the incapacity of the individual, and the level of informal support (from family and friends) which is available to them. For an individual, there are three important characteristics: physical ability (mobility and the ability to carry out daily living tasks); mental ability (dementia or behavioural disorder); and incontinence. Different combinations of these will generate different service requirements.

The role of informal support is much more difficult to assess, but it does have an important mediating effect on whether, or to what degree, statutory services provision becomes involved. Informal carers often absorb much, if not all, of an individual's social care requirements, and their presence or absence will have a significant impact on the response demanded of other – formal – services.

Table 8.4 is an example of how dependencies of different kinds are used to make up a classification. Each combination of dependencies, such as 'severe physical disability' and 'moderate incontinence' and 'no mental disability' and 'good informal support', defines a dependency group. Even with only three scale points for each dependency there are $3 \times 3 \times 3 \times 3 = 81$ possible dependency groups. However, in real populations many combinations are not found and generally between 10 and 20 groups will be sufficient.

**Table 8.4** An example of dependency categorization

|  | Conceptual dimension | Examples of scale categories | | |
|---|---|---|---|---|
|  |  | 'Normal' | Moderate | Severe |
| 1.1 | physical disability | ambulant | chairbound | bedbound |
| 1.2 | mental disability | normal | confused | dementia |
| 1.3 | incontinence | continent | urinary | faecal |
| 2 | informal support | good | occasional | poor |

For each category, a variety of packages of care can be considered. For example, people with severe physical disability, moderate incontinence and no dementia might be cared for on a geriatric ward or in a residential home (Table 8.5).

**Table 8.5** Potential care options for a specific dependency category: severe physical disability, moderate incontinence and no dementia

| Service Care options | Option 1 | Option 2 | Option 3 | Option 4 |
|---|---|---|---|---|
| Geriatric ward (wks/yr) | 52 |  |  |  |
| Residential home (wks/yr) |  | 52 |  |  |
| Day hospital (attendances/wk) |  |  | 2 |  |
| Home visits (hrs/wk) |  |  | 5 | 5 |
| Home help (hrs/wk) |  |  | 12 | 16 |
| Preference order | 2 | 4 | 1 | 3 |
| Annual cost (£) | 7190 | 1230 | 3669 | 1760 |

Notice that the definition of each package of care includes the types of resources involved and standards as to the amount of each type. The different packages of care for any given dependency group may be given preference rankings but all the packages should be acceptable. Definition of the dependency groups, the corresponding packages of care, their preference rankings and the resources implied provide the structure of the model.

The next step is to gather information on, or estimate, first, the numbers of people in the population in each dependency group, and, second, the amounts of each relevant resource available. With regard to numbers in each dependency group, there may be good local data to hand. But more commonly estimates have to be made based on methods similar to the ones you learned about in Chapter 7. Age- and sex-specific rates from surveys in other populations can be applied to the local population structure.

Cropper and Forte (1997) provide practical guidance on obtaining data on resources and using the model.

###  Obtaining data for the Balance of Care model

In principle, information on the quantity, location and cost of services is more straightforward to obtain. In practice, however, data are often held by different agencies in different systems (not all of which are computer-based), and there may be different data definitions to contend with as well. While it can be inconvenient to assemble the data, nonetheless it is usually possible to do so. The BoC system, importantly, aids this process first by focusing attention on data relevant to the planning issues; second, it enables people to progress in their planning without having to wait for every item of data to be gathered and verified. It is very easy to enter data into the system, so initial estimates or 'best guesses' for data items can always be used to start with and updated as time goes on . . .

The system comprises two principal components: a population model, and a care options model. The population model . . . uses a combination of census data and dependency data collected in a previous Balance of Care project survey (the 'base district') to generate estimates in 16 different dependency categories for any given locality. The system enables the user to . . . explore alternative assumptions about [local levels of informal support] based on local knowledge.

A number of simple, built-in routines allocate the population of a particular dependency group to care options automatically on the basis of specified preferences or lowest cost, but the user can also specify individual allocations either in conjunction with the automated routines or completely independently of them.

The system provides analyses of the care options across all dependency groups showing, for example, how the cost consequences of a particular scenario impact on dependency levels or on funding or provider agencies. Implications for the quantities of particular services are also provided, both in total and by individual dependency group. Users can start, therefore, by obtaining an overall impression of the potential impact of a particular scenario, and then gradually zoom in on this view to see how it affects individual dependency groups or services. This enables assessments to be made of the appropriate mixes of services in terms of service levels, costs, and how they relate to dependency and locality within the study area. At this point authorities have to reconcile conflicting objectives of cost efficiency and service effectiveness, and take into account other constraints which may be imposed by existing patterns of service delivery and manpower. It is possible to return to the care options or allocations, make adjustments as desired and recalculate the results in a matter of seconds. Users can thus enter an iterative cycle of testing assumptions until they are satisfied that any strategic objectives and constraints have been recognized.

 **Activity 8.8**

Gibbs (1978) says that 'by providing a set of connecting logic between service inputs and intermediate outputs, the model may enrich the quality of the planning dialogue between central and field authorities'. Describe this 'connecting logic', as you understand it from the extract from Cropper and Forte (1997).

 **Feedback**

The logic of the model is essentially as follows:

1 Define a set of *dependency groups* of patients that are similar to each other in terms of their *needs for care*.

2 For each dependency group:

   (a) develop alternative modes of care, defined by *packages* of resources (some better than others, but all acceptable);
   (b) estimate *numbers* in the group to be found in the population served.

3 For each mode or package of care:

   (a) identify the resources involved;
   (b) agree *standards* – how much of each resource is needed for each mode;
   (c) agree *preferences* – rank the different modes for each group in terms of desirability.

4 For each *resource*:

   (a) determine *costs* per unit of resource used;
   (b) identify *constraints* in terms of how much of each resource is available (upper limit) and/or what must be used (lower limit).

5 Identify performance *criteria*. The Balance of Care model uses:

   (a) *coverage* – proportion of dependency group receiving any appropriate care package;
   (b) *quota* – numbers with preferred service;
   (c) *numbers* with any service.

This is illustrated by Table 8.6, which is based on a recent version of the Balance of Care model. It shows the kinds of information needed on modes, standards and preferences. As in Table 8.1, the different kinds of resource are listed down the left-hand side, but otherwise Table 8.6 is laid out rather differently because Table 8.1 only dealt with one dependency group: patients needing surgery on their varicose veins.

**Table 8.6** The balance of care model: groups, modes, standards, preferences

| Service | Service Units | Unit of Measure | £ Gross cost per unit | Current service levels | Dependency group 2 Care Options n = 124 | | | | Dependency group 4 Care Options n = 376 | | | | | | Dependency group 12 Care Options n = 50 | | | | | |
|---|---|---|---|---|---|---|---|---|---|---|---|---|---|---|---|---|---|---|---|---|
| | | | | | Hospital long stay | Geriatric Day Hospital | Private Nursing Home | Government Nursing Home | Hospital long stay | Psychiatric Day Hospital | Home | Private Nursing Home | Day Centre | Government Nursing Home | Residential Accommodation | Day Centre | Sheltered Housing | Health Visitor | Private Residential Home | Psychiatric Day Hospital |
| Long stay ward | Beds | wks pa | 350 | 300 | 52 | 24 | | | 52 | 10 | 10 | | 10 | | | | | | | |
| Psychiatric long stay | Beds | wks pa | 400 | 80 | | | | | | | | | | | | | | | | |
| Day hospital | Places | days pw | 86 | 75 | | 1.5 | | | | | | | | | | | | | | |
| Psychiatric day hospital | Places | days pw | 125 | 45 | | | | | | 2.4 | | | | | | | | | | 3 |
| Community nurse | WTE | hrs pw | 34 | 130 | | | | | | 0.8 | 1.6 | | 2 | | | | | | | |
| Comm. psych. nurse | WTE | hrs pw | 38 | 10 | | | | | | 1.2 | 1.2 | | 2 | | | 2 | 2 | 2 | | 2 |
| Health visitor | WTE | hrs pa | 49 | 2 | | | | | | | | | | | | 8 | 17 | 8 | | |
| Domiciliary physiotherapy | WTE | hrs pm | 34 | 6 | | | | | | | 2 | | 2 | | | | | | | |
| Private res. home | Beds | wks pa | 185 | 600 | | | | | | | | | | | | | | | 52 | |
| Private nursing home | Beds | wks pa | 280 | 175 | | | 52 | | | | | 52 | | | | | | | | |
| LA residential accom. | Beds | wks pa | 252 | 980 | | | | | | | | | | | 52 | | | | | |
| Sheltered housing | Beds | wks pa | 10 | 1500 | | | | | | | | | | | | | 50 | | | |
| Day centre | Places | vsts pw | 25 | 94 | | | | | | | | | 3.2 | | | 2 | 2 | 2 | | 2 |
| Home help | WTE | hrs pw | 7.7 | 300 | | 5 | | | | 7 | 10 | | 6 | | | 4 | 4 | 4 | | 4 |
| Domicil Care assistant | WTE | hrs pw | 15 | 90 | | 11 | | | | 11 | 11 | | 11 | | | 10 | 10 | 14 | | 8 |
| Night sitter | WTE | nts pm | 70 | 0 | | 4 | | | | 3.2 | 4.8 | | 3.2 | | | 3 | 3 | 3 | | 3 |
| Domicil occup. therapy | WTE | hrs pa | 20 | 15 | | | | | | | 6 | | | | | | | | | |
| Meals on wheels | Meals | mls pw | 3 | 1400 | | 1.5 | | | | 2 | 4 | | 2 | | | 3 | 3 | 5 | | 2 |
| Domiciliary laundry | Sets | sets pw | 2 | 0 | | 3 | | | | 1 | 1 | | 1 | | | 1 | 1 | 1 | | 1 |
| Govt Nursing home | Beds | wks pa | 290 | 125 | | | | 52 | | | | | | 52 | | | | | | |
| Preference indicator | | | | | 1 | 2 | 4 | 3 | 5 | 1 | 3 | 0 | 2 | 4 | 2 | 3 | 4 | 5 | 0 | 1 |

Note: WTE = whole time equivalent; wks = weeks; hrs = hours; mls = meals; pa = per annum; pw = per week; pm = per month.

In a Balance of Care model there may be up to 40 groups, the upper limit depending mainly on:

- the extent to which it is possible to distinguish usefully between dependency groups;
- the effort involved in defining the alternative modes for each group.

The model has 16 groups but in Table 8.6 information is given for only three (dependency groups 2, 4 and 12).

- For each group, Table 8.6 gives the number of people in the population served. This may be based on primary survey data or estimated by applying age–sex specific rates from studies elsewhere to the demographic structure of the local population.
- For each group there are several columns, each representing a possible mode of care for the group in question.
- For each mode there is a figure against some of the resources listed on the left; these represent the package of resources necessary for the appropriate standard of care in that mode.
- At the bottom of the column for each mode there is a preference indicator which represents a consensus judgement about the relative desirability of the mode. Thus for dependency group 2, hospital long-stay ward is the most preferred option; geriatric day hospital, nursing home, and patient's home follow in that order.

The shaded area gives information about the costs of each unit of resource and current levels of provision. This allows modelling to be carried out subject to constraints defined by upper budget limits and current resource levels. In other 'what if' scenarios, budget limits and resource levels may be varied.

 **Activity 8.9**

The following extract from Forte and Bowen (1997) describes how this kind of model has been used as a basis for planning workshops.

As you read this, make notes on:

1  How you would summarize the points and arguments in favour of its use at the local level as an aid to planning care of the elderly.
2  What you think might be some of the problems and weaknesses.

 **Improving the balance of elderly care services**

Past experience has demonstrated that the take-up of the system from cold – that is, without any additional support – is relatively poor. The workshop programme . . . has been developed not as a simple 'system tutorial' but as a means of demonstrating the potential of the BoC approach in a real application using local data and issues as its focus and directly engaging local planners, managers and professionals.

The workshop helps to reinforce the development of links between local agencies by bringing together key players, and by recognizing and accommodating the importance of each of their contributions: this applies not just across organizations, but across disciplines as well. Having someone familiar with the computer system to facilitate the workshop means that attention can be focused during the workshop on addressing the planning issues themselves.

In one workshop . . . the first chapter comprised an initial demonstration of the model to a group of about 40 people so there could be a wider understanding of the overall aims of the workshop and what their core group colleagues would be addressing in future chapters. Planning issues, data sources and responsibilities were also identified for subsequent stages.

The second chapter took place a few weeks later when the core group [of 16 people] reassembled for an intensive two-day chapter. Sub-groups were formed to consider the demographic and dependency characteristics of the elderly population as estimated by the model as well as information on current service levels and costs drawn from a variety of local sources. The task of translating care policies – published and otherwise – into service implications with respect to dependency levels was led by a consultant geriatrician. This is the central feature of the approach: getting people to focus on appropriate quantities and types of service with respect to different dependency char-acteristics, and trying to move away from the strong bias which tends to exist towards service-based planning (i.e. basing future plans on existing patterns of service and facilities).

While this work was under way, data, planning assumptions and ideas were continually entered into the system by the group facilitator. Gradually, the resource implications began to unfold over the two days as data and planning ideas were entered, their effects calculated and opinions revised and refined. The computer screen was projected onto a screen so all participants could see the results immediately, make 'real time' suggestions to try out different assumptions and watch them analysed instantly. This method of working was very fruitful; many more ideas could be tested out than would have otherwise been the case with an equivalent paper-only exercise. A lot of debate was stimulated which, apart from focusing on the results, also brought to light all sorts of questions about data sources, namely their accuracy, how they could be improved, and where there were obvious gaps. At the end of the second day an action plan for taking forward the main points emerging was drawn up and a copy of the model, data and print-out left with the Social Services Department.

The third chapter of the workshop took place about two months later with a presenta-tion of the model and local results to a group of operational-level health service staff including community nurses and residential home managers. In the interim, people had already started to refine their ideas and to think about translating the exercise from the county to a locality basis; most importantly, they had gone on to use the model for themselves without further external support. This was an important outcome, as a key aim of this workshop programme is not just to provide a 'one-off' event, but to get the principles of the approach more firmly embedded into the routine local planning and contracting process. Several months later the outcomes of the workshop were infor-mally reviewed with some of the participants. A number of positive effects were cited, ranging from input to the development of a respite care policy to staff training. The participative nature of the workshop was found to provide a good way of involving operational care provider staff directly in the planning process, particularly through the focus on needs assessment and the discussions around the specification of care options where their operational-level knowledge was particularly valuable. Moreover, the approach was felt to complement the work of established planning structures while, at the same time, adding more rigour to the use of existing information (and highlighting inadequacies where they occurred).

In more general terms the workshop was also acknowledged to have helped strengthen relationships between planning authorities. The BoC system provided a strong focus for this. Even where it did not provide an 'answer', it contributed significantly to a clearer understanding of the underlying components of planning problems by exposing hitherto implicit assumptions about data and aspects of policy. The ability to incorporate user and carer ideas and preferences was also appreciated.

Inevitably there were difficulties in assembling data and agreeing assumptions to be made. Apart from the all-important local commitment, the approach requires an intensive time input during the workshops to be effective. Some thought also needs to go into tailoring the model for particular local circumstances, for example, considering what different care options might be required for different ethnic groups. Ultimately, though, the fact that it took this effort and time is not a fault of the approach itself but rather a recognition of the complexity of the issues involved.

*Concluding remarks*

An important feature of [decision support systems] like the Balance of Care system and approach, is their ability to enable users to gain insights into the overall resource consequences of policy directions, and to pave the way for further, more detailed work which will often fall outside its immediate scope.

The structure of the computer system is such that it can maximize the use of any additional information which is locally available from surveys or other data sources and that it can be used at different levels of sophistication appropriate to the particular problems faced locally. Some authorities, for example, have found it useful simply as a starting point for looking at ways of improving existing local information on dependency levels and service utilization, and have found that a demonstration and group discussion of the model is sufficient in itself to stimulate ideas. Others have gone on to a more detailed examination of care policies, quantifying care options and substituting local data where available as outlined in the examples above. There are no hard-and-fast rules as to what constitutes an 'application'; this will vary across districts and with local priorities.

The idea of an applications workshop within which the most recent BoC system version is used has been the most significant development in trying to ensure that users of the system can exploit its full potential . . . With the first release of the microcomputer system it was expected that managers would be able to use it directly themselves without much in the way of applications support. Subsequent experience has suggested that the model is better understood with initial support and so the idea of integrating it with a facilitated workshop – which is much more than a system tutorial – came about.

'Would the same approach work in my area?' The short answer is yes. However, no decision support system or workshops can substitute for a lack of local commitment to the planning process by any of the key players. Nor can BoC – or any other [decision support system] succeed easily if there are constant problems in continuity caused by the constant ebb and flow of reorganization and people changing jobs and responsibilities. All organizations blame each other at one time or another for the lack of progress; unfortunately although this has long been recognized to be unhelpful, it continues to happen today.

The Balance of Care approach and system cannot give perfect answers to complex strategic planning issues at the push of a button and was not designed to do so. However, it does make a good starting point for the development of strategic thinking and action. Where a robust joint planning framework is already active, it can highlight areas of potential development for effective solutions and help to present them in more imaginative ways. As the quality and quantity of the information base for community services increase, so does the potential to tackle short-term planning and organizational issues. The BoC system can be used to support such activity and stimulate the move towards better local information systems.

## Feedback

1 Arguments in favour of using the Balance of Care model at the local level.

Perhaps the most widely recognized strength of the model lies in its logic and structure. This has provided a framework for:

(a) bringing together the many different agencies and professions involved in providing long-term care for elderly people and stimulating substantive discussions about how to define dependency groups and alternative modes of care for each group;

(b) taking population needs, rather than particular resources or services, as the starting point for planning;

(c) pulling together and organizing existing information, and identifying needs for additional information.

The fact that the model runs fast on a personal computer has the advantages of:

(d) *responsiveness*. Once the model has been set up, it is possible to evaluate a range of planning scenarios quickly; thus it is possible to try out a planning idea, look at the results, and make successive revisions until a satisfactory balance is achieved.

(e) *portability*. The model can be used in different people's places of work; results can be projected onto a large screen, so that there can be widespread participation in the planning process, which is desirable when so many agencies are involved.

2 Potential problems and weaknesses.

These fall into two categories: problems with data and problems with the process. Problems with data include the following:

(a) Collecting local primary data can be costly and time-consuming. If data collection takes a long time, this can lead to planning blight in which even the most obvious planning decisions are not made because the decision makers are 'waiting for the model'.

(b) The model provides age- and sex-specific rates for each of the dependency groups from several representative areas. These can be applied to the demographic structure of the local population to get round the need for local data. But very little is known about the accuracy of estimates based only on these two factors and how much real needs vary from one area to another.

(c) In practice, each additional case cared for in a particular mode will not involve the same marginal cost. However, the model's linear approach to cost estimation ignores effects such as returns to scale and cost triggers (such as opening a new ward or taking on an additional member of staff). Arguably this is more of a problem with using the model for local than for regional or national planning.

Problems with the process include:

(d) Meetings required for real collaboration are time-consuming; senior staff may not give the necessary time; juniors may not have the necessary authority to commit their organization to any resulting plans.

(e) Any model of this kind requires estimates of the amounts of resources necessary to provide care of an acceptable standard within each mode. Although experience with the model suggests that it is generally possible to establish a consensus on this, there can be difficulties, particularly if there is a lack of goodwill or if certain provider agencies are trying to gain an advantage.

It is commonly argued that as a basis for providing care for individuals, these groups are too crude; two people in the same group could have very different needs for care. But this is a planning tool, not a set of treatment guidelines. As Cropper and Forte (1997) observe:

At the operational level it is important to ensure some degree of choice [in the package of care for each individual], but at the strategic level of service commissioning the issue is to establish the broad direction for service provision.

The approach has also been criticized because it does not explicitly address questions about the impact of decisions on the effectiveness of care. However, for services such as care for incontinence or confusion, questions about effectiveness are less relevant than they might be for acute care. Also, as Gibbs argued in 1978:

In most public services the relationship between intermediate and final outputs is not well understood. Although it is right that long-term research should be undertaken where there is a reasonable chance of elucidating the relationship, the modeller who is currently involved in strategic planning has to provide answers now. He must therefore formulate his model in terms of intermediate or proxy measures as best he can. He should not feel inadequate in doing this. The information gap between intermediate and final outputs is not a problem for him alone; it is also a problem for all those involved in strategic planning whether they use mathematical models or not.

Finally, in the first part of this chapter you learned about linear programming. This method was originally designed to provide best solutions to problems that involved many different kinds of resources and constraints but now it is not used in that way. Here is another extract from Gibbs (1978):

The use of optimizing models normally depends upon a formal quantitative statement of the objectives of the system being modelled. In public services agreed statements of this type are difficult, if not impossible, to obtain. Thus it will usually be necessary, as was the case with the Balance of Care study, to formulate a simulation type of model. (Although the algorithm used in the Balance of Care model is of the optimizing type, the model is of the simulation type in the way it is used – the user specifies a set of resource levels and the model simulates how the service will respond.) One special merit of such a model is that, because it is normally used iteratively, the customer for the model has a good opportunity to understand how the model works. As the customer gains a deeper knowledge of the model assumptions he may wish to modify some of them to accord with his understanding of the system. This is a double gain for the model – it improves the assumption structure and it gives the customer more confidence in using the model.

There is still a great deal to be learned about the relationship between health care activity and outcomes, and a lack of clarity about health care objectives. Although Gibbs was writing nearly 30 years ago, his points are still valid. With changing technology and contested values, they are likely to remain so.

## Summary

In this chapter, you have learned about linear programming as an approach to the question of how to achieve a good mix or balance of service provision, given service and budgetary constraints and minimum requirements.

You went on to read about an approach to planning services for elderly people that has constraints linear at its core. This allows decision makers to explore the pros and cons of different configurations of resources in an interactive way, but perhaps just as importantly it can provide structure to the processes of gathering and interpreting information and coordinating the roles of different providers.

## References

Cropper S and Forte P (eds) (1997) *Enhancing Health Services Management*. Buckingham: Open University Press.

Forte P and Bowen T (1997). Improving the balance of elderly care services, in S Cropper and P Forte eds. *Enhancing Health Services Management*, pp. 71–85. Buckingham: Open University Press.

Gibbs RJ (1978) The use of a strategic planning model for health and personal social services. *Journal of the Operational Research Society* 29: 875–83.

Tramarin A, Tolley K, Campostrini S and Lalla F (1997) Efficiency and rationality in the planning of health care for people with AIDS: an application of the balance of care approach. *AIDS* 11: 809–16.

# 9 Hospital models

## Overview

Decision support systems are widely used in the hospital sector to assist in planning activity and budgets. In this chapter you will learn about the interrelation between activity changes and costs and then examine the use of a hospital model to forecast activity in an acute care setting. You will consider multiple linear regression as a modelling technique that can process aggregate data from many hospitals to identify predictors of cost and then look at case mix models that are based on detailed data from hospital management information systems.

## Learning objectives

By the end of this chapter, you will be better able to:

- identify different types of cost and explain how they change with activity
- discuss alternative approaches to estimation of hospital costs
- outline the use of a hospital model in activity and capacity planning
- interpret and use models based on multiple linear regression
- give examples of alternative approaches to modelling hospital costs
- explain the use of DRGs in hospital management

## Key terms

**Diagnosis related groups (DRG)** Classification system that assigns patients to categories on the basis of the likely cost of their episode of hospital care. Used as a basis for determining level of prospective payment by purchaser.

**Fixed cost** A cost of production that does not vary with the level of output.

**Flexible budget** A budget showing comparative costs for a range of levels of activity.

**Semi-variable costs** Costs that contain both a fixed and a variable element.

**Total (economic) cost** The sum of all costs of an intervention or health problem.

**Variable cost** A cost of production that varies directly with the level of output.

## Introduction

Hospital planning models are decision support systems for the hospital sector. They are mainly used in hospitals that operate in a contractual environment to provide reliable information for business planning. Modelling can be applied to the following areas:

- financial monitoring and planning: to provide analysis and estimates of hospital speciality costs at a given activity level and to forecast the cost consequences of changes in resource or activity levels;
- hospital service planning: to forecast consequences of changes in activity for staffing, beds, operating theatres, etc.

This is a complex task, as changes in service provision cause cost changes and changes of costs of inputs may influence activity levels. You will therefore first examine the relationship between cost and activity and then look at an example of a model for forecasting activity levels and different approaches to modelling hospital costs.

## How do hospital costs behave?

Costs can be defined as measures of loss of monetary value when a resource is acquired or consumed (Perrin 1988). This definition suggests that costs are not just cash flow. A monetary loss may not only occur when a resource is *acquired* but also while it is *consumed*. Some resources are used up quickly and frequently such as stocks, consumables and staff time or labour. Other resources are used slowly over the long term, such as buildings and equipment. The important thing is for hospital managers to be aware of how the costs of using different resources relate to activity so that it is possible to anticipate this.

If you are able to assess costs for various levels of activities, then you are in a position to:

- forecast and budget;
- calculate prices for the services in a contractual environment;
- compare costs between wards, specialities or hospitals;
- determine whether a service should be provided in-house or contracted out.

Health services require many different types of resources, such as building, equipment, staff, drugs and consumables. The costs of a specific service depend on:

- the resources employed (the resource mix);
- the quantity of each resource required.

By definition, all resources incur a cost when they are employed. If the level of activity stays constant, costs won't change. If activity goes up, costs will change but the extent to which this happens is not straightforward. Resources have different characteristics in the way their costs are affected when activity changes. The way in which costs respond to changes in activity is called cost behaviour.

### Different types of costs

How much a service costs at different levels of activity depends on the cost behaviour of its inputs. You need to group the resources into broad categories according to how their consumption changes with activity. These categories are variable, fixed, semi-variable and stepped costs:

- *Variable costs* change simultaneously with activity in a linear relationship. When output increases, costs go up when output decreases, costs go down. This linear relationship can be defined algebraically by:

  $y = bx$

  where y = cost, b = variable cost and x = level of activity.

- *Fixed costs* stay constant (in the short run) with changes in activity. Fixed cost resources must be acquired and fully functioning before any output can be produced but their costs not increase as output increases. The function is:

  $y = a$

  where y = cost and a = constant.

- *Semi-variable costs* contain a fixed and a variable element. These resources incur a standing charge that is payable regardless of whether the input is used plus a cost that varies as activity increases. This relationship is represented by the linear equation:

  $y = a + bx$

  where $y$ = total cost, a = fixed cost element, b = variable cost element and x = level of activity.

- *Stepped costs* behave like fixed costs but only until a certain threshold is reached. When activity increases further, costs step to a higher level. This process continues as output increases.

### Activity 9.1

Categorize the following resources of a health centre into fixed variable, semi-variable and stepped costs:

drugs, doctors, telephone, X-ray equipment, consumables, laboratory assistant, appliances, general manager, building, nurses, X-ray plates

### Feedback

| | |
|---|---|
| Fixed: | X-ray equipment, general manager, building |
| Variable: | drugs, appliances, consumables, X-ray plates |
| Semi-variable: | telephone |
| Stepped: | doctors, nurses, laboratory assistant |

### Total cost

Total cost is the combination of all these resources at a certain level of output. If you know how costs behave, you can summarize the cost for each type to work out total cost at a given level of activity. This approach is useful in preparing a flexible budget, as you will see in the following activity.

 **Activity 9.2**

An environmental health laboratory is performing 1000 analyses per year. Its income was £60 per analysis in the last year. The Ministry of Health wants to increase the number of analyses from next year. The equipment is fairly new and runs well below its capacity but sample processing is labour-intensive and one laboratory assistant can handle up to 1000 analyses per year. The average salary of a laboratory assistant is £15,000 per year. You are asked to set up a flexible budget for 2000, 3000 and 4000 tests per annum, based on the information in Table 9.1.

**Table 9.1** Various budget costs for tests 1

| Number of tests | Fixed costs | Stepped cost | Variable cost | Total costs | Total income | Balance |
|---|---|---|---|---|---|---|
| 1000 | 100,000 | 15,000 | 1300 | | 60,000 | |
| 2000 | | | | | | |
| 3000 | | | | | | |
| 4000 | | | | | | |

 **Feedback**

Preparing a flexible budget requires you to identify the income and cost outcomes for the different potential levels of activity. You should have arrived at the numbers in Table 9.2.

**Table 9.2** Various budget costs for tests 2

| Number of tests | Fixed costs | Stepped cost | Variable cost | Total costs | Total income | Balance |
|---|---|---|---|---|---|---|
| 1000 | 100,000 | 15,000 | 1300 | 116,300 | 60,000 | −56,300 |
| 2000 | 100,000 | 30,000 | 2600 | 132,600 | 120,000 | −12,600 |
| 3000 | 100,000 | 45,000 | 3900 | 148,900 | 180,000 | 31,100 |
| 4000 | 100,000 | 60,000 | 5200 | 165,200 | 240,000 | 74,800 |

The activity shows the importance of fixed costs in management decisions. If you have a fixed cost problem, you should consider cutting these (which can be difficult) or, if they are unavoidable, to increase activity levels to spread the fixed costs more widely.

### Average and marginal costs

In addition to total cost, you may also look at average and marginal costs. Average cost is calculated by dividing total cost by the quantity produced:

TC/Q

## Activity 9.3

Work out the average cost for 1000, 2000, 3000, 4000 tests in the example above.

## Feedback

1000 = £116

2000 = £66

3000 = £50

4000 = £41

As you see in this example, average costs are initially high because fixed costs are spread over a small output. As output rises, fixed costs are spread over more and more tests, reducing the average costs.

Marginal costs are the cost for producing one more unit of output, for example, the extra cost of moving from four tests to five tests. This can be calculated using the following formula:

ΔTC/ΔQ

where ΔTC is the change in total costs and ΔQ is the change in the quantity of outputs.

Marginal costs are useful in incremental analysis. These are the costs a manager needs to assess in business planning. For example, what does it cost to treat 10 more patients? In a simple example, with just fixed cost and variable cost, marginal costs are equivalent to the increase in variable cost as output rises.

The calculation gets more complicated when semi-variable and stepped costs are considered. As health services are complex, there may be a large numbers of cost factors that change with activity. Think, for example, of the knock-on effects for support services if activity increases. It can get difficult to calculate the cost function for any given level of activity and here computer-based hospital models can assist.

## Using hospital models in projecting costs and planning of services

One of the challenges for hospital managers is how to project the impact of changes in activity on financial performance. During the planning cycle the budget is prepared based on estimated levels of activity, and when comparing actual results with the budget, you need to estimate again what the costs should have been for the actual levels of activity which were achieved. Hospital models can assist in the planning process but like any model they provide a simplified representation of reality and their predictions and estimates are bound to be approximations. Costs are difficult to predict because health care is highly complex and varies with patient needs which cannot be perfectly predicted. Despite these limitations, quantitative models are an important source of information. They increase the analytical capabilities of an organization and assist managers in decision making.

The crucial point of any hospital model is the quality of data that are used as inputs and the degree to which it takes account of the interaction between different variables. Hospital models have been used for activity and capacity planning (Beech et al. 1990; Bowen and Forte 1997). They can integrate data that are already available and take account of the links and interdependencies between different parts of the organization.

## An example of capacity planning: the business planning model

One particular challenge of publicly funded health systems is the management of waiting lists for access to specialist care. Models have been used to monitor the implementation of goals for reduction of waiting times.

In Bowen and Forte's (1997) business planning model, the main components are based on an iconic model with boxes and arrows to display service pathways. The upper part displays activity and waiting lists, the lower part the use of resources (Figure 9.1).

Any approach to reducing waiting lists has resource implications. The additional costs of reduced waiting times are often related to changes in staffing requirements. Calculation is based on stocks and flows of patient numbers. In practical terms the model was first developed as a 'paper' model with only some of the key variables such as occupancy rates, length of stay and numbers of patients seen as day-cases. Managers of all specialties were involved in providing the data. The model was then refined and developed further by producing a prototype spreadsheet version which included all the variables in the flow diagram.

Different scenarios can be explored by changing a range of parameters in the model. In the specific hospital under investigation, this suggested that doing nothing would lead to a steady increase in waiting lists. If only the in-patient waiting list were reduced, the outpatient waiting list would continue to rise. And if only the outpatient waiting list were reduced, the in-patient waiting list could rise substantially. Achieving service targets with given levels of resources involved a balance between activity levels in the different service areas.

Before introducing such a model you need to have clear management objectives, related to agreed levels of service provision, the required activity to achieve these targets and possible efficiency gains. It is also important to organize a learning process in which all participants are enabled to develop their analytical skills and to gain ownership of the model. All users need to understand how the model works, what adjustments can be made and how it is updated.

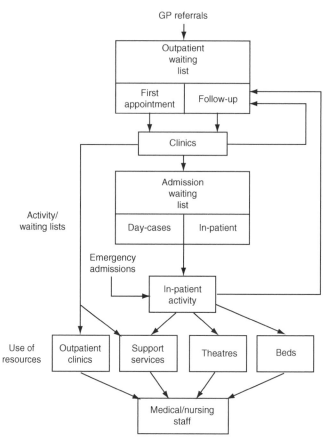

GP referrals

**Figure 9.1** The business planning model
Source: Bowen and Forte (1997).

## Multiple linear regression

Capacity models deal with activities and capacities but do not predict costs. One approach to estimating costs is to use aggregate data from different hospitals, typically from the routine hospital data systems. Multiple regression is a statistical technique that can be used to estimate the influence of a range of variables on total cost. For example age, severity of disease, presence or absence of co-morbid conditions and length of stay may all be predictive of patient costs. The multiple regression equation is of the form:

$$y = a + b_1x_1 + b_2x_2 + c_2x_3 + \ldots$$

where y might be the average cost per patient episode, $x_1$, $x_2$, $x_3$, etc. the variables used to predict costs, and $b_1$, $b_2$, $b_3$, etc. the *partial regression coefficients*. Normally a statistical computer package such as SPSS or Stata is used to estimate these coefficients, together with standard errors and confidence intervals, p values for significance tests and $R^2$ for the amount of variance explained.

Söderlund and colleagues (1997) took routinely collected cost and activity data for 638 acute hospitals in the UK to estimate the effect of trust status, competition, and the mix of purchasers on average hospital costs per in-patient, after adjusting for outpatient activity levels, case mix, teaching activity, regional salary variation, hospital size, scale of activity, and scope of cases treated (Table 9.3). Note that some of the independent variables have been expressed as indices. For example, the authors used indices based on ordinal scales for case mix, wages and level of specialization. 'Trust status' refers to the organizational status of the hospital after separating purchasing and providing in the 1990s. In this context, competition as measured by the market concentration index had no influence on costs.

**Table 9.3** Multiple regression analysis assessing factors influencing average cost per in-patient episode

|  | Coefficient | 95% Confidence interval | | P value |
|---|---|---|---|---|
|  |  | Lower | Upper |  |
| Intercept | −699.39 | −988.86 | −409.92 | 0.0001 |
| Case mix index | 9.25 | 7.99 | 10.51 | 0.0001 |
| Long stay days/in-patient | 5.31 | 3.07 | 7.54 | 0.0001 |
| % of multiple episodes | −6.46 | −11.59 | −1.32 | 0.0140 |
| Outpatient attendances/in-patient | 22.97 | 8.63 | 37.32 | 0.0018 |
| Accident and emergency attendances/in-patient | 35.57 | 1.24 | 69.89 | 0.0427 |
| Day attendances/in-patient | 325.80 | 259.21 | 392.40 | 0.0001 |
| Student whole time equivalents/in-patient | 88266 | 64845 | 111687 | 0.0001 |
| Capital price index | 31.89 | −10.69 | 74.48 | 0.1427 |
| Wage price index | 2.53 | 1.65 | 3.40 | 0.0001 |
| Inverse of in-patient episodes | 2742914 | 1886546 | 3599282 | 0.0001 |
| Average number of beds | 0.19 | 0.11 | 0.28 | 0.0001 |
| Specialization index | 102.45 | 42.32 | 162.58 | 0.0009 |
| Trust status | −38.80 | −84.89 | 7.28 | 0.0994 |
| Market concentration index | 15.71 | −97.94 | 129.36 | 0.7865 |

Source: Söderlund et al. (1997).
Notes: Sample size = 638 hospitals; adjusted $R^2$ = 0.07.

## Hospital models as part of the information technology system

While multiple regression modelling is suitable for economic and health policy analysis, the method is rarely used in individual hospitals. A hospital manager who is concerned with tactical service planning needs to answer questions such as:

- If a service is expanded by a certain amount, how many extra beds and theatre sessions will be required?
- What will it cost?

Hospital models that can help answer these questions are part of the hospital information technology (IT) system in high income countries. These computerized systems have been introduced since the late 1980s enabling hospitals to improve their performance through better information management. They can manage large amounts of data and are capable of providing timely information needed for many management decisions. IT can combine the areas of accounting, patient administration, procurement, and human resources management. These areas can be linked to case mix information and provide managers with information for monitoring, controlling and decision making. Thus IT-supported hospital models can provide timely information about how much a service costs and what factors affect its costs. However, there are some drawbacks:

- A system for collecting activity and cost data needs to be in place. The additional recording and reporting can cause problems as it is not always welcomed by clinicians when it puts additional pressures on them. Advanced systems have bedside computer terminals and portable data entry devices which allow activity to be recorded in real time.
- Hospital information systems are expensive, not only in terms of hardware and software but also in terms of staff training and maintenance. Hospitals operate in a rapidly changing environment and software needs to be updated frequently to account for changes in clinical practice, management policies and purchasers' demands.
- Hospital models are useful in a contracting environment where providers have to deal with different forms of payment and different purchasers. Models can be designed to fit into the general management accounting system. If groups of hospitals use the same system, performance can be compared across hospitals and consolidated reports can be produced. IT is still prohibitively expensive for many low income countries but basic solutions for budgeting and forecasting are increasingly being introduced.

## Cost triggers

Cost triggers are an important feature of hospital planning at the local level. As activity levels increase, some costs (such as pharmaceuticals perhaps) may increase in proportion but capital and equipment costs may be stepped or 'lumpy'. A piece of equipment or ward may have a particular capacity. As long as activity levels are within that capacity, capital costs are fixed. But to expand activity levels beyond current capacity involves additional capacity and extra cost, such as building a new ward or opening one that is out of commission. Similarly, reducing capacity may not save much in the way of costs unless the reduction is enough to close a ward or dispose of an item of equipment.

Beech and colleagues (1990) developed a hospital planning model with input data taken from routine sources. Outputs include financial as well as service planning data. Service planning outputs allow the feasibility of changes in activity levels to be assessed. Are there enough beds to achieve target flow rates? Is there enough theatre capacity to increase the number of operations? Financial planning outputs include changes in costs that result from changes in activity levels and the sale or acquisition of capital.

In such a model the approach to costing cannot be based on average costs because these are not closely enough related to changes in activity. Beech and colleagues use the marginal approach to costing, with cost triggers such as links between patient admission rates and opening or closing wards and between the number of operating sessions and opening or closing theatres. Any model of this kind has to be tailored to the local situation and this can involve substantial effort in surveying opinion and collecting data.

## Case mix systems

More advanced models record activity for each patient. Their common element is a case mix (*patient classification*) system that allow the types of patient treated to be related to resource use. They usually incorporate information on diagnoses, procedures and severity of disease. A range of further dimensions can be included so as to model the course of treatment, such as intensity of care (e.g. low dependency, high dependency, intensive care), type of admission (e.g. in-patient, outpatient) and the time spent in hospital.

One commonly used system is *Diagnosis Related Groups* (DRGs), which was developed at Yale University in the 1980s and first used in reimbursing providers of treatment for Medicare patients in the USA (Fetter et al. 1980). Since then the model has been refined and adapted to different uses and settings. DRGs are now used in the management of hospitals in several high income countries and a range of middle income countries have tried them. Although for managers, the main function of a case mix system is to provide the basis for prospective case-based payment of hospital services, they are also being used for a range of other purposes such as:

- *research*: a classification system such as DRGs can provide detailed information on service use for clinical and health services research
- *planning*: a number of countries use case mix systems for strategic capacity planning and contracting for the hospital sector. In population level models, case-mix information is used to simulate costs and consequences of changes in service provision, such as a move to an essential package of health care.
- *resource allocation*: case mix systems are used in a number of countries to allocate and devolve central budgets
- *quality improvement*: patient classification systems support the development of clinical pathways and guidelines and allow the performance of health care organizations to be compared across a wide range of inputs and outputs.

In the past decade DRGs have become increasingly popular as a basis for prospective payment for hospital services. A DRG allows a fixed price to be set for all cases in the same diagnostic category. Purchasers can set the reimbursement level to the average cost for each DRG and the hospital is usually free to decide on the number of cases treated, the inputs used and length of stay.

Under this system providers have strong incentives to increase efficiency by offering services at a near to or below average price (Donaldson and Gerard 2005). Hospitals may, for example, seek to make a surplus by delivering the service with shorter lengths of stay, by specializing in certain treatments, by substituting inputs or through economies of scale.

### The approach

Typically a DRG system used for financial management combines information from the following sources:

- patient data (demographic and clinical, such as age, sex, diagnosis, co-morbidity and complications);
- activity data (on types of procedures and interventions received, length of stay);
- financial data (cost profiles per individual case or agreed cost weights).

Each case is assigned the appropriate diagnostic and procedural category as well as dimensions that capture and differentiate the process of care. The latter may include a range of variables such as sex, age, length of stay, mental health, legal status, birth weight and hours of mechanical ventilation.

The way each case is assigned to the correct DRG is determined by an algorithm, a detailed sequence of instructions describing the method for doing a task which ensures accuracy and efficiency of data processing. For example, in the Australian DRG system the code consists of the following three distinct elements which are connected in a logical sequence and worked through in the coding of each case:

- the main diagnostic category (MDC), based on the WHO International Classification of Diseases;
- the type of treatment received – medicine or surgery;
- the level of resource use, based on an index measuring clinical complexity and co-morbidity of the case.

As the model is meant to provide a realistic representation of the treatment process, the quality of coding is paramount. Each DRG has a unique code describing the diagnosis and course of treatment. For example, in the code B70A (for stroke with severe complications), the letter B refers to the MDC and signifies that the DRG belongs to the broad category of disorders of the nervous system, the figure 70 specifies the diagnosis/procedure, here stroke with medical treatment, and the letter A signifies the highest level of resource use out of four categories A–D.

## Attaching costs to DRGs

Every DRG is linked to a cost weight which reflects the resource use according to disease severity and the complexity of the procedures employed. Usually the average cost across all DRGs is chosen as a reference value, which is called the *base rate*. For example, if the base rate is $2000 and the actual average cost for treating a case with a specific disease is $4000, then a cost weight of 2.0 will be attached to this DRG, as the cost of treatment is double the cost of an average case. DRGs with a resource use below average have a cost weight < 1, above average of >1.

The cost weight takes account of the actual input needed for treating a case. For example, a complicated case of appendicitis will attract a relatively high cost weight of 2.02, to reflect the longer hospital stay after appendectomy. The income/price (I) for this case would be

Cost weight × base rate = I
2.02 × £2000 = £4040.

In contrast, if the cost weight for an uncomplicated appendicitis is 1.09, the hospital would receive only 1.09 × £2000 = £2180.

Table 9.4 shows an example of four adjacent DRGs for patients in a stroke unit, reflecting different reimbursement levels according to case complexity and resource use. As you can see, for the hospital it is particularly important to capture the correct level of disease severity as much of the hospital income depends on correct coding. Increasingly, this job is done by skilled coders who review medical records for the assignment of the correct DRG. Where several thousand cases have to be processed, coding is supported by an analytical software tool, a so-called grouper.

**Table 9.4** Four adjacent DRGs of a stroke unit

| DRG | Text | Number of cases | Cost weight | Average LOS (d) | Reimbursement per case ($) |
|---|---|---|---|---|---|
| B70A | Stroke with catastrophic complications/co-morbidity | 10 | 1.78 | 10,7 | 2670 |
| B70B | Stroke with severe complications/co-morbidity | 25 | 1.389 | 11,5 | 2084 |
| B70C | Stroke without severe or catastrophic complication | 35 | 1.169 | 9,8 | 1754 |
| B70D | Stroke, patient died within four days of admission | 2 | 0.654 | 2,4 | 981 |

### Activity 9.4

As you have seen, case mix models can be used for service planning as well as for financial planning. If a case-mix management system is used by your organization, list the information on which it is based. Alternatively, if you do not have a case-mix management system, think how you would design one, listing the information that would be needed. In either case, your answer should be structured under three headings:

1  Patient information needed.
2  Activity information needed.
3  Financial information needed.

### Feedback

1 Patient information may include demographic data (sex, age, insurance status), main diagnosis, co-morbidity, complications and level of disease severity.

2 Activity-related information includes procedures performed, length of stay, in-patient/outpatient treatment and theatre use, number of outpatient attendances.

3 Financial information includes cost per day, cost per outpatient attendance, cost of specific procedures such as mechanic ventilation or dialysis, or the agreed cost weights attached to each case if a DRG system is used for reimbursement.

## Monitoring case mix

Internationally, DRG systems and the approaches to monitoring case mix vary widely. Some countries use only 20 DRGs, others more than 800. To be able to negotiate prices, managers need good information about the costs and case mix of the services provided.

Base rates calculated for individual hospitals can be used to compare cost per case across a region or the entire country. The *regional base rate* is important in a competitive environment as it can be used by purchasers to set prices. Providers whose base rate is below the regional average will have a competitive advantage, while those with a base rate higher than the regional average will make a loss.

A tool that is frequently used for this is the case mix index (CMI). The CMI is a measure of average disease severity across all cases treated in an entire department or hospital during a year. Take, for example, a department with only two types of DRGs: 100 cases were treated with a relative weight of 2.02, and 50 cases with a relative weight of 1.09. Then the CMI is calculated as follows:

$(100 \times 2.02) + (50 \times 1.09) = 256.5$ which is divided by the total number of 150 cases
$256.5/150 = 1.71$.

As a clinical department will have many more than just two types of cases, the calculation is applied to all DRGs used in the department. The CMI allows annual income to be assessed. Similarly the departmental CMIs can be combined into one CMI for the entire hospital:

Income from DRGs = number of cases × CMI × base rate

Using DRGs for modelling hospital costs is complex and expensive because it involves exact information about the costs per case and careful monitoring of the case mix. While a DRG system offers strong incentives to use resources efficiently, it can also be linked to negative effects. A range of measures are usually taken to avoid or minimize these:

- Case mix models should capture the course of treatment accurately but not support bad clinical practice. The model should be built on agreed guidelines and clinical pathways. Its use should be accompanied by rigorous audit to ensure quality of care. Also, DRGs should be updated yearly to reflect changes in clinical practice or the introduction of new technologies.
- Pricing systems based on DRGs will usually make a range of provisions to discourage unwanted provider behaviour, particularly under-provision of services and inappropriate admissions and discharge. In a competitive environment under-provision can arise when expected case numbers are small and thus relatively expensive to treat. This may occur in remote rural areas and additional incentives are usually given to run hospitals in these regions. Inappropriate admissions and early discharge may occur when the provider expects that the costs of a specific case are under-recovered.
- Another set of challenges is related to coding of cases. Because disease severity, complications and co-morbidity attract higher cost weights, providers will tend to keep the CMI at a high level. Inappropriate coding of cases, inadvertently or deliberately, is not uncommon and patients may thereby appear sicker than

they are. This form of misclassification, which is called DRG creep, leads to unjustified reimbursement levels. In response purchasers will monitor changes of the CMI carefully and review records of selected cases (Nowicki 2001).

## Summary

You have seen how hospital models can assist in financial monitoring and service planning. They can be used to forecast speciality costs at a given activity level and, vice versa, to forecast the consequences of changes in activity for inputs such as staffing, beds and theatres. Awareness of how costs behave is essential for understanding hospital models. Multiple regression analysis allows identification of predictors of cost and modelling of cost components based on information from many hospitals.

You have considered the hospital planning model which uses routine data and the marginal costing approach, based on cost triggers. Case mix models record activity for each patient based on systems that allow the type of patients treated to be related to resource use. As a key example of a case mix model you examined the purpose, use and limitations of DRGs in hospital management.

## References

Bailey TC and Ashford JR (1984) Speciality costs in English hospitals: a statistical approach based on a cost component model. *Journal of the Operational Research Society* 35: 247–56.

Beech R, Brough RL and Fitzsimmons BA (1990) The development of a decision-support system for planning services within hospitals. *Journal of the Operational Research Society* 41: 995–1006.

Bowen T and Forte P (1997) Activity and capacity planning in an acute hospital, in Cropper S and Forte P (eds) *Enhancing Health Services Management*. Buckingham: Open University Press.

Donaldson C and Gerard K (2005) *Economics of Health Care Financing: The Visible Hand* (2nd edn). Basingstoke: Palgrave Macmillan.

Fetter R, Shin Y, Freeman J, Averill R and Thompson J (1980) Case mix definition by diagnosis-related groups. *Medical Care* 18(2): 1–53.

Gruen RP, Constantinovici N, Normand C and Lamping DL for the North Thames Dialysis Study (NTDS) Group (2003) Costs of dialysis for elderly people in the UK. *Nephrology Dialysis Transplantation* 18: 2122–7.

Nowicki M (2001) *The Financial Management of Hospitals and Healthcare Organizations* (2nd edn). Ann Arbor, MI: Health Administration Press.

Perrin J (1988) *Resource Management in the NHS*. London: Chapman & Hall.

Söderlund N, Csaba I, Gray A, Milne R and Raftery J (1997) Impact of the NHS reforms on English hospital productivity: an analysis of the first three years. *British Medical Journal* 315: 1126–9.

# SECTION 4

# Modelling for evaluating changes in systems

# Modelling flows through systems

## Overview

In Chapter 1 you learned to distinguish between models representing effects (or influences), logical stages and flows. You were also introduced to system models, which involve both influences and flows. In this chapter and the next you will learn about a number of approaches to modelling systems. Such models can play useful roles in analysing the possible outcomes of different policy options.

In the first part of this chapter you will learn how flows through systems can be represented using simple 'tree' models. These can be useful for questions about the routes that flows of patients may take as they move through the system, if 'outcomes' can be measured at a fixed time after intervention. But if outcome events are spread out over time and can occur more than once, another approach may be needed. In the second part of this chapter you will learn about Markov models.

Another important issue is whether the situation in some 'downstream' parts of a system affects flow rates 'upstream'. The nature and extent of any such feature of a system, called 'feedback', can determine how the system as a whole behaves, and in the third part of the chapter you will learn more about this. Finally, you will learn about the limitations of modelling flows as flows, rather than the sum of the experiences of individuals. In Chapter 11 you will learn about modelling the experiences of individuals, known as microsimulation.

## Learning objectives

**By the end of this chapter, you will be better able to:**

- use representations of flows, states, events and influences to describe the performance of systems
- use tree structures to model flows through a system
- explain the Markov property and Markov chains
- explain the role of system dynamics and feedback in complex system behaviour

## Key terms

**Feedback loop** The causal loop formed when flow rates out of a process or state influence the flow rates into it.

> **Markov process** An approach to modelling how systems behave over time based on the assumption that the probability of an object moving from one state to another in a given time period depends only on what the initial and final states are, and not on the object's 'history' of events or time spent in the initial state.

## A tree model of a smoking cessation programme

In Chapter 6 you learned to use tree structures to represent decision problems. The examples were about specific decisions facing individuals, such as how to treat a particular patient and decisions about how many operating theatres to build at a particular hospital. In this chapter you will start by using a tree model to address a policy issue.

There is good evidence that nicotine replacement therapy (NRT) can help people stop smoking. Imagine that your government is thinking about encouraging its use but there are concerns about the cost-effectiveness of such a programme. You have been asked to build a model that will provide estimates of the likely cost per quitter (person stopping smoking).

The sort of programme that is being proposed would involve the following:

* People known to be smokers are given brief advice by their primary care doctor and invited to participate in a cessation programme.
* All participants have a programme of counselling and are prescribed one month's supply of NRT.
* Some people will drop out quite quickly but those who complete the first month are prescribed a second month's supply of NRT.

On the basis of your discussions with policy makers, you carry out a literature search from which you derive the estimates for probabilities and costs in Table 10.1. One useful source is the health technology assessment by Woolacott and colleagues (2002).

**Table 10.1** Data for the NRT quit-smoking model

| Probabilities | | Mid (%) | SD (%) | Costs | | Mid (£) | SD (£) |
|---|---|---|---|---|---|---|---|
| p1 | agreeing to participate in the programme | 20 | 6 | c1 | Brief advice | 4.00 | 1.00 |
| p2 | participants adhering to the programme | 50 | 10 | c2 | Counselling | 36.00 | 6.00 |
| p3 | adherers quitting | 10 | 3 | c3 | NRT 1st month (all participants) | 37.00 | |
| p4 | non-adherers quitting | 7 | 2 | c4 | NRT 2nd month (adherers only) | 37.00 | |
| p5 | non-participants quitting | 3.5 | 0.50 | | | | |
| p6 | quit rate without programme | 2.0 | 0.30 | | | | |

Note: 'Quitting' means being a non-smoker one year after the beginning of the programme.
Source: adapted from Woolacott et al. (2002).

**Activity 10.1**

1 Using a spreadsheet, set up a tree model. As well as the probabilities for each branch, show the numbers in a target population of 1000 smokers who would be expected to 'flow' down each branch. (You can use the word 'quit' as shorthand for 'a non-smoker one year after the beginning of the programme'.)

2 Estimate the costs and benefits to the health care system of offering the programme to 1000 smokers compared to not offering it.

 **Feedback**

Figure 10.1 (see over) shows a version of the model, with the numbers flowing down each pathway. In the area at the bottom of the figure is a simple two-branch 'comparator' tree which shows what would happen if there were no NRT programme.

The 'results' section of the model shows the numbers at the end of each branch and where the costs fall. The total marginal cost of the programme is £22,300 for 1000 smokers. Of the 1000, 45 would be expected to quit if there were a programme. Without the programme, 20 would be expected to quit, so the marginal benefit is 25 quitters at a cost of £22,300.

You can see that the costs of such a programme would be around £892 per quitter. To examine the calculations, open the file 'Ch10Prev' and have a look at the spreadsheet called 'Tree'.

### Sensitivity analysis

With this simple model, a sensitivity analysis can be done using the standard deviations in Table 10.1. The idea is that there is some uncertainty around the 'mid' estimates, which can be represented by distributions possible values with their means at the 'mid' estimates. In this case the assumption is that the distribution are Normal, so that the probabilities of the true values being more than 2 standard deviations higher or lower than the 'mid' estimates are both around 2.5 per cent.

The results of the sensitivity analysis are set out in the range A43:S47. In this range, cells C45 to H45 allow you to sample values for each probability and cost in the model in such a way that if you repeat the analysis many times the distribution of sampled values for each input parameter will be Normal, with the mean and standard deviation specified in 'Data'. With a zero in row 45, the 'mid' estimate for the parameter in question is used in each calculation, but with a 1 in this row, a different sampled value is used each time. In the area A48:S2047 the calculation of cost per quitter is repeated 2000 times. This is called the Monte Carlo technique, and you will learn more about how it works in Chapter 11.

The mean and standard deviation of the 2000 calculations of cost per quitter are given in cells S46 and S47. Because of the sampling process the actual figures will be different each time the spreadsheet is recalculated, but if all the parameters are sampled, the mean estimate of cost per quitter is around £950, with a standard

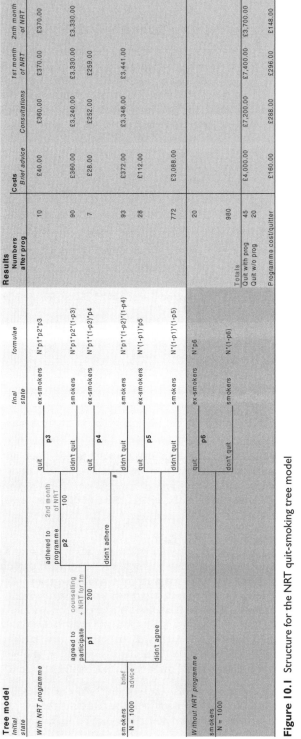

**Figure 10.1** Structure for the NRT quit-smoking tree model

deviation of around £400. This means that given the levels of uncertainty about the input parameters there is a lot of uncertainty about the 'mid' estimate for cost per quitter. The results are particularly sensitive to uncertainty about the value of p5.

Notice that the mean cost per quitter using sampled values is higher than it is using 'mid' values. The *median* cost per quitter over the 2000 samples is very similar to the 'mid'-based estimate though. This is because the distribution of the cost effectiveness ratio is not symmetrical, but skewed to the right. The denominator of the cost per (additional) quitter is the difference between the numbers of quitters with and without the programme, and in some samples this difference will be very small. Also if you press F9 to resample, you will find that the standard deviation of the cost per quitter is very variable with 'only' 2000 replications each time.

### Estimating health benefits

This may seem helpful in broad terms but it doesn't allow for direct comparisons with other possible health care programmes. This requires estimating the numbers of years of life saved. To do this with a simple tree model you have to make some fairly gross assumptions. The paper on smoking among male British doctors by Doll and colleagues (2004) suggests that, on average, long-term quitters gained around 3, 6, 9 and 10 years of life, depending on whether they gave up at around age 60, 50, 40 or 30. However, in the analysis by Woolacott and colleagues (2002) it was assumed that on average the benefit of quitting was living only two years longer. Depending on which assumption is right, the crude cost of NRT per year of life saved could be anything between about £300 and £500.

The picture is complicated by the fact that in most evaluations of policy, benefits and costs are *discounted*. Years of life saved will 'arrive' earlier in some programmes than in others, and will in general be valued more highly, and so will be discounted less. Also the benefits from giving up smoking are different for women and men, and for people of different ages. Thus the cost-effectiveness of the programme will depend on the structure of the local population of smokers.

However, the most damaging criticism of a simple decision tree approach to this particular problem is that smoking habits are subject to continuous change. Quitting is not a once-and-for-all event; ex-smokers may start smoking again, or 'relapse'. Equally, quitting does not *only* occur as a result of this programme. People who quit during the programme might well have quit anyway a few years later. If so, the true contribution of the programme would be a few additional smoking-free years, rather than decades. To make reasonable estimates of health benefits, these factors need to be taken into account. A third problem with this kind of model is that it would be very unusual for such a programme to be offered just once. In a real programme, known smokers might be invited to participate once every few years.

To summarize, simple tree models can be helpful if the exposure or intervention is followed by the events or outcomes of interest *within a specific time horizon*. Tree models have been used to analyse strategies for prenatal screening, for example. In smoking cessation a simple tree model might be used for estimating programme costs per programme quitter if quitting is defined as being a non-smoker at some specific time after the intervention – say, one year, as in Activity 10.1. However, such models may be misleading if the times from intervention to a relevant outcome are uncertain (such as quitting outside the programme, relapsing or the onset of a smoking-related disease), or if some patients experience the intervention several times over or undergo several changes of state.

One way of overcoming this is to divide the period during which relevant events might occur into a series of shorter periods or cycles. The distribution of outcome events can then be modelled by stringing a series of trees together, each tree showing the numbers of events during a defined period. Each cycle should be short enough to allow the assumption that each individual will experience at most one event per cycle.

Such an approach would lend itself to evaluating a cyclical prevention programme. If it were proposed that smokers would be eligible every five years, a basic model could involve a five-year cycle. Figure 10.2 illustrates this for three cycles.

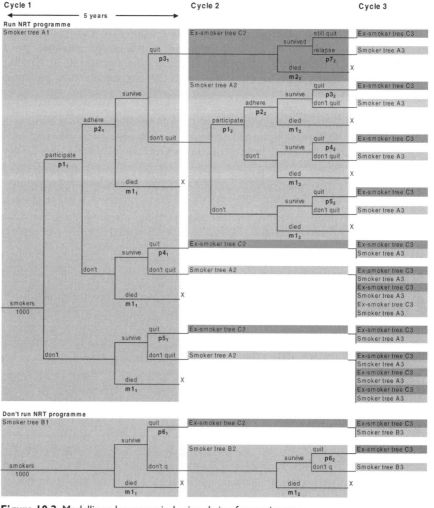

**Figure 10.2** Modelling a longer period using chain of recursive trees

Notice that:

1 This diagram is composed of three basic trees, used recursively, i.e. the ends of branches in one cycle can become 'trunks' for similar trees in the next cycle. The trees for smokers in populations with an NRT programme (smoker tree A) and for smokers in populations with no such programme (smoker tree B) are almost identical in structure to those in Figure 10.1. However, there are also trees for ex-smokers in the second and all subsequent cycles, because you are interested in whether they relapse and become smokers again. This means data are needed on relapse rates, shown in Figure 10.2 as p7.

2 In the simple tree model the probability of death within the period modelled was ignored, but for five-year cycles this becomes important. So now as well as 'smoker' and 'ex-smoker' there is a third possible state: 'died'. This allows you to model the health effects of the programme by using different death rates, shown in Figure 10.2 as m1 for smokers and m2 for ex-smokers. In each case the 'died' branch splits off after the 'participate' and 'adhere branches' because costs will be attached to flowing down these branches and it is assumed that the intervention programme is at the beginning of the cycle before significant numbers have died. The 'died' branch splits off before the 'quit' branch because most of the data on quitting are rates for survivors.

3 The structures of the corresponding trees in each cycle are the same. Smoker Tree A in the first and second cycles branches in the same way. (Smoker Tree A in the third cycle is also the same but there is not enough space in Figure 10.2 to show its structure.)

4 You can use different sets of probabilities and mortalities in each period (e.g. $p1_1$ to $p6_1$, $m1_1$ and $m2_1$ in the first period, $p1_2$ to $p7_2$, $m1_2$ and $m2_2$ in the second period etc.). This is important because the probabilities of quitting and relapsing may vary with age, and mortality rates will certainly increase. To make this clear, tree A is labelled 'Tree A1' in cycle 1, 'Tree A2' in cycle 2, etc.

For Smoker Tree A there are three routes through to each of the three *states*, i.e. nine final branches. Each of the three branches that ends in 'smoker' provides the starting point for another 'smoker' tree in the next cycle, and the three branches that end in 'non-smoker' each become another non-smoker tree. The branches that end in 'died' go no further, as this is an 'absorbing' state with no flows out. Thus in each cycle, each smoker tree branches into six further trees. It is clear from Figure 10.2 that the number of branches can become very large and the tree can become 'bushy' and unwieldy. In this case the basic tree has few branches and only three cycles are involved. You can imagine what such a model might look like if the basic tree had 20 branches and there were 20 cycles.

## The Markov property

The model can be simplified quite dramatically by making one simple but far-reaching assumption. If you could describe the three groups of the people who were still smokers at the end of period 1 – those that had been through the entire programme, those that had been through part of it and those who had not participated at all – as being essentially interchangeable for the purposes of the model, you would need only one smoker tree in the next cycle instead of three – and also only one in period 3 instead of 12, etc. You could do the same for all those who ended period 1 in the 'ex-smoker' category. Then each period would start with just one smoker tree and one ex-smoker tree and there would be no 'spreading' of the tree at all.

This is illustrated in Figure 10.3. Each cycle consists mainly of a version of the smokers' tree (Figure 10.1) with 'died' branches added. At the end of each cycle the numbers of ex-smokers, smokers and deaths are pooled and used as 'inputs' to the next cycle.

In this diagram $s0_1$ is the number of smokers at the beginning of period 1, $s1_1$ is the number of smokers coming out of the 'adhere' branch in cycle 1, $e1_1$ the number of ex-smokers and $d1_1$ the number of deaths, etc. All you need from each tree in each period is the total number of outcomes of each type, shown in Figure 10.3 as e.g. $e1_1$ $+ e2_1 + e3_1$ for the total numbers of ex-smokers at the end of cycle 1. From this tree you can work out that the numbers of ex-smokers at the end of cycle 1 is

$e1_1 + e2_1 + e3_1$ where
$e1_1 = s0_1{}^*p1_1{}^*p2_1{}^*(1 - m1_1){}^*p3_1$
$e2_1 = s0_1{}^*p1_1{}^*(1 - p2_1){}^*(1 - m1_1){}^*p4_1$
$e3_1 = s0_1{}^*(1 - p1_1){}^*(1 - m1_1){}^*p5_1$

In subsequent cycles the people who gave up in earlier cycles and are still ex-smokers will have to be added in, so the number of ex-smokers after cycle 2 becomes e.g. $e1_2 + e2_2 + e3_2 + e4_2$, etc.

What is the implication of this assumption? When you merge all the streams at the end of each cycle you *lose information* – or 'forget' – about the route that each person took through the series of cycle-trees up till that point. This does not matter if the route does not affect the probabilities in future periods. However, one might expect that, for example, someone who had a long history of failed attempts at giving up smoking would have relatively poor prospects of success in the future. Also, someone who gave up smoking many years ago has a lower risk of death than someone who has only just quit. With a 'memoryless' model we would not be able to take such factors into account.

The key assumption is that the probability of moving from state X to state Y in a given cycle can be treated as being the same for everyone who was in state X at the beginning of the cycle and independent of what happened in the past. This means that it is independent of:

• the number of people who started the cycle in state X. This would not be true if smoking were essentially a social phenomenon, for example. If it were, the more people who smoked, the more difficult it would be to give it up, and the smaller the probability of making the transition from smoker to ex-smoker.
• the states that they have been through in previous cycles. This would not be true if having been a smoker for a long time meant it was more difficult to give up.

This kind of model is called a Markov process after Andrei Andreyevich Markov (1856–1922), a Russian mathematician. In short, the Markov or 'memoryless' property means that the probability that an object moves from one state to another in a given time period depends *only* on what the initial and final states are.

Suppose that a proportion, $p_{se}$ of the people who were smokers at the beginning of a cycle will be ex-smokers at the end of it and a proportion $p_{sd}$ will die. Also $p_{ed}$ of those who were ex-smokers at the beginning of the year will have died by the end

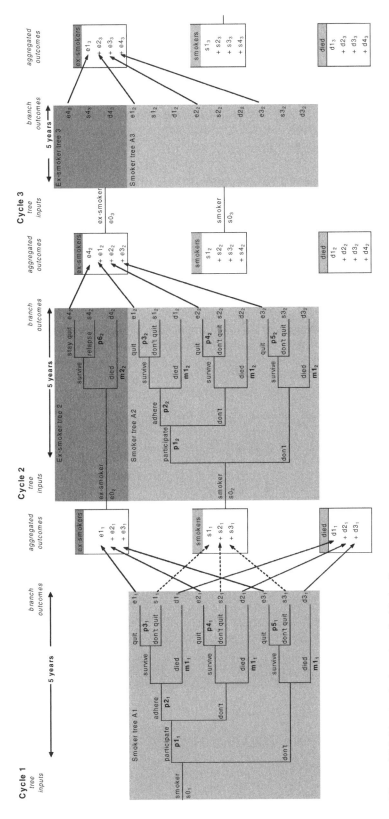

**Figure 10.3** Merging the branches of a 'chained' tree

| At time T | At time T + t |  |  |
|---|---|---|---|
|  | smoker | ex-smoker | dead |
| smoker | $1 - p_{wi} - p_{wd}$ | $p_{se}$ | $p_{sd}$ |
| ex-smoker | $p_{es}$ | $1 - p_{es} - p_{ed}$ | $p_{ed}$ |

**Figure 10.4** A transition matrix

of it. Finally, $p_{es}$ of the patients who were ex-smokers at the beginning will be smoking again by the end. From these states and proportions (called *transition probabilities*) you can construct a *transition matrix* like Figure 10.4.

If you can assume the Markov property and know the current state of the system, you can use this set of transition probabilities to work out the expected flows between states, and thus how many people are smokers, ex-smokers and dead at the end of cycle 1. Then, rather like the computation of a life table, you can take the numbers in each state at the end of cycle 1 and use the set of transition probabilities to work out the numbers in each state at the end of cycle 2. By repeating this process you can work out the numbers in each state at the end of cycle 3, 4, 5 . . . 10, and so on. Figure 10.5 illustrates the position at the beginning, at the end, and at some intermediate point in such a process.

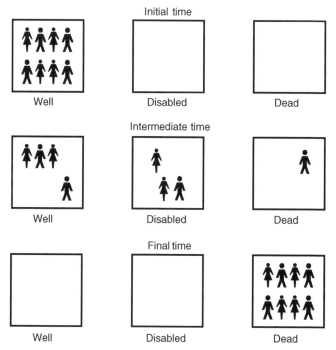

**Figure 10.5** A Markov process
Source: Sonnenberg et al. (1993).

If the number of states involved is finite and the transition probabilities do not change over time, this is called a Markov *chain*. Markov chains can be 'solved' by matrix algebra to give the expected survival time in each state under different conditions. However, in many health care applications it is important that the transition matrix should be able to change with the passage of time, usually because one of the states is death or onset of disease, and the risks of these change as people grow older. Such problems are commonly modelled using spreadsheet software.

## A Markov model of the smoking cessation programme

Now try using this method to evaluate the smoking cessation programme. Look at 'Markov 5yr' in the file on your CD called 'Ch10Prev'.

In the yellow (data) area on the left are the probabilities. Overall these are consistent with the probabilities that you used in your simple tree model but since the cycle length is five years, whereas the quit rates in the simple model were for after one year, an adjustment has been made to allow for smokers quitting and non-smokers relapsing in the remaining four years. (If you are interested, the calculations are given on the spreadsheet called 'Prob estimates'.)

This model is for a cohort of 1000 men, all of whom are 40 years old at the beginning of the analysis. The probabilities in a model of this kind will change as the people in the cohort grow older, so the layout of Table 10.1 has been turned on its side and broken down by age group. This in turn allows you to bring in some additional information from the literature, which suggests that:

- of those who do try to give up smoking, older people are more likely to be successful than younger people;
- older smokers are less likely to volunteer for smoking cessation programmes than younger ones.

Probabilities of death for smokers and ex-smokers are based on the data from Doll and colleagues (2004) given in Table 10.2. These are rates for men and so the model will be for men, although there is some evidence that the benefits of quitting are greater in women. Note that Doll's figures suggest greater benefits from quitting than some other studies, so the results may be favourable to quit-smoking programmes. The yellow data area also contains costs and discount rates, which will be explained shortly. (Although this model is based broadly on the literature, it has to be relatively simple for learning purposes and should not be used for 'real' policy analysis!)

Next is a slim green area headed 'control variable'. This allows the model user to determine which age groups should be included in the programme. Currently there is a 1 in P8 and zeros in the other cells in column P. This means that only people in the age group 40–44 would be eligible, i.e. there would only be one intervention cycle per cohort. If all these zeros had been ones, each person in the cohort would have been eligible to participate every five years.

The 'model' is in the rust-coloured area. On the left is a transition matrix that has been derived from the data in the yellow area. The key to this is the long expression

**Table 10.2** Overall mortality among never smokers, ex-smokers, and continuing cigarette smokers in relation to stopping smoking at ages 35–64, for men born 1900–1930 and observed during 1951–2001

| | Annual mortality per 1000 men | | | | | | | | | |
|---|---|---|---|---|---|---|---|---|---|---|
| | Life-long non-smokers | | Ex-cigarette smokers, by age stopped | | | | | | Continuing smokers | | Mortality ratio smoker vs non-smoker |
| | | | 35–44 | | 49–54 | | 55–64 | | | | |
| Age range | rate | n | rate | n | rate | n | rate | n | rate | n | non-smoker |
| 35–44 | 1.6 | 55 | – | | – | | – | | 2.7 | 150 | 1.6 |
| 45–54 | 3.3 | 145 | 5.4 | 95 | – | | – | | 8.5 | 487 | 2.3 |
| 55–64 | 8.4 | 290 | 9.0 | 132 | 16.4 | 229 | – | | 21.4 | 703 | 2.5 |
| 65–74 | 18.6 | 528 | 22.7 | 262 | 31.7 | 331 | 36.4 | 250 | 50.7 | 722 | 2.7 |
| 75–84 | 51.7 | 666 | 53.1 | 316 | 69.1 | 370 | 78.9 | 299 | 112.2 | 453 | 2.2 |

Source: Doll et al. (2004).

in cells U9, U11, etc., which is essentially the formula given above for numbers of quitters in a cycle, derived from the cycle tree in Figure 10.3. The other formulae correspond to those in Figure 10.4.

The model is set up to simulate a cohort that continues through 11 cycles until the survivors complete their 95th year. The table on the right of the rust-coloured area shows the state of the system at the beginning and end of each cycle. It shows that of the initial cohort of smokers (X9 = 1000), by the end of the first cycle about 110 are ex-smokers since the transition probability from smoker to ex-smoker after five years for this age group is 0.110 (see cell U9). Also about 19 of the 1000 smokers (X9*V9) have died, the transition probability of smoker to death after five years being 0.019 in this age group (in cell V9). This leaves 870 smokers (X11) and 110 ex-smokers (X12) to start the second cycle. And so on.

## Activity 10.2

1   Copy formulae to fill in the blanks in the rest of the 'State of the system' table in 'Markov 5yr'.
2   With an NRT programme for those aged 40–44 only, how many smokers and ex-smokers are alive at the beginning of the 9th cycle?

## Feedback

1   At the beginning of the 9th cycle there are 146 smokers and 188 ex-smokers still alive.
2   The table should look like the corresponding one in the spreadsheet called 'Markov 5yr 2'.

### Calculating and comparing costs and benefits

'Markov 5yr 2' has a number of additional features. First of all, two programmes (A and B) are provided for. This will allow you to compare the cost-effectiveness of programmes involving different target age groups.

Second, there is a new pale blue area on the right called 'Results'. Column AE simply shows the number of deaths during the cycle. In column AF this is converted into a number of life years lived during the cycle by assuming that, on average, deaths occur mid-way through the cycle. Thus, with 1000 people starting cycle 1 and 19.13 deaths after five years, in cycle 1 there are $(1000 - 0.5*19.13)*5 = 4952.18$ years of life. Column AG shows the difference in life years in each cycle between Programme A and Programme B.

Column AH shows the cost of running the programme in each age group/cycle. This is calculated from the probabilities and costs in the yellow area.

Both costs and life years are discounted by the rates given in the yellow data area. This is done by dividing the costs arising in each cycle by $(1 + \text{discount rate})^{(\text{discount years})}$, using the discount years in column AD.

Cell AG3 at the top of the blue area shows the cost-effectiveness ratio derived from a comparison of Programme A and Programme B. This is calculated as the difference in costs of the programmes, discounted as appropriate, with and without the programmedivided by the difference in discounted years of life lived by the cohort with and without the programme.

### Activity 10.3

Now you can use this model to investigate the cost-effectiveness of different types of programme.

1 Compare a programme for which those in age group 40–44 are eligible, with no programme. What is the cost-effectiveness of the programme in terms of £ per year of life saved? How does this compare with the results from your tree model? Why do you think they are different?

2 What happens to the cost-effectiveness ratio if your programme involves intervening in every cycle, i.e. every fifth year?

3 Now, staying with intervention every fifth year, try discount rates of 3 per cent for costs and 3 per cent for benefits. What does this do to the cost-effectiveness ratio? Why do you think this happens?

4 Do you think that modelling in five-year periods is too long, too short, or about right?

### Feedback

1 Since only those aged 40–44 are eligible, a '1' is placed in cell P8, and the rest of the cells in column P for programme A are zero or blank. All the cells in column P for programme B are zero or blank. With no discounting, the cost of programme A per

year of life saved is £546. Doll and colleagues suggest that quitting permanently at age around 40 would give nine extra years of life, and if it were assumed that quitters in the simple tree model do not relapse, this would suggest a cost of around £892/9 = £99 per year of life (YoL) gained. This seriously underestimates cost per YoL, and thus over-estimates cost-effectiveness, mainly because many quitters *will* relapse after a year of non-smoking. Using the figure of two years of life saved per quitter at one year, which somehow takes subsequent relapses into account, brings the estimates more into line.

2 £494 per year of life saved, so the programme has become slightly more cost-effective. In fact, the programme is slightly more cost-effective in the 50–69 age range than in the 40–44s because of the higher quit rates and lower relapse rates, but less so above about 70 because the programme costs the same per participant in these older men, but the average number of years of life saved is less. You can check this by looking at the effects of intervention in specific older groups.

3 £1004 per year of life saved. The programme is less cost-effective with discounting because the costs are incurred at the time of the intervention but the benefits mainly come later. You can see this by looking at the ages at which life years are saved in column AG. Thus the costs are discounted less than the benefits. Discounting always disadvantages disease prevention programmes when compared to acute treatment programmes.

4 Too long. One problem is that new quitters do not have their death rates reduced until the cycle *after* they have changed 'state'. Thus someone who quits smoking at age 41 does not have their risk of death altered until they are 45. The result is under-estimation of the benefits of intervention. Also the model assumes only one event per cycle. If someone gives up smoking at age 41, say, but relapses at age 44, they are counted in the model as being a smoker for the whole cycle. If an ex-smoker relapses at age 41 and quits again at age 44, they would be counted as ex-smokers throughout, which means that the model over-estimates the benefits. This mixture of over- and under-estimation of benefits makes it very difficult to say whether the model over- or under-estimates cost-effectiveness overall. This is quite a common problem with such models.

## A one-year cycle model

In Ch10Prev there is a spreadsheet called 'Markov 1yr'. The shorter cycle length requires a much larger spreadsheet but makes more direct use of the published data on quitting and relapsing, which are typically one-year rather than five-year rates. The preliminary calculations in 'Prob estimates' are unnecessary, although the assumptions are the same. Also in many studies of the effectiveness of smoking cessation, subjects are only counted as having quit if they are still non-smokers after one year, so the assumption of only one 'event' per cycle is more reasonable.

The risks of death and background quit and relapse rates in the five-year model are adapted for a one-year cycle in e.g. H8:K8 by using the formula

1-year % = 1 − (1 − 5-year %)$^{1/5}$

The numbers of deaths per cycle in this model are lower than in the five-year model and the numbers who quit and relapse higher, as you would expect.

In this model the corresponding answers to those for Activity 10.3 are: £529, £433 and £913 per year of life saved. The figures are lower than those from the five-year model in each case because the five-year model under-estimates the benefits more than the one-year model. The under-estimate is greatest in the programme with intervention in each five-year age group because the error arising from delaying reduction of new ex-smokers' death rates until the following cycle arises in every group.

 **Activity 10.4**

In the light of the data from Doll and colleagues in Table 10.2, do you think that using a Markov model is a reasonable approach to this problem?

 **Feedback**

One important feature of Doll et al.'s results is that the benefits of smoking cessation depend both on the person's age and on how old they are when they quit. However, in this simple Markov model the risk of death for ex-smokers depends only on their age. It would be possible to build a Markov model that allowed for both factors but it would involve *disaggregation*, i.e. splitting the 'ex-smoker' state into age-specific substates, such as 'ex-smoker, quit between 35 and 44', 'ex-smoker, quit between 45 and 54', etc. In this way risks of death could be applied that also depended on age at quitting.

## Pros and cons of Markov models

The advantages of Markov models over tree models are that:

- the effects of repeated intervention and repeated changes of state can be modelled;
- interventions (implying costs) and changes of state (implying benefits) take place within given time periods so that costs and benefits can be discounted;
- risks and probabilities can change with the passage of time or, equivalently, with the ageing of a cohort, which can be important in the context of health care.

Like tree models, Markov models can be built using standard spreadsheet software and there are add-ins available such as @RISK, which allow parameter values to be sampled from distributions rather than remaining fixed. If there is uncertainty about the actual model input parameter values, this technique can provide an indication of the uncertainty surrounding the model outputs.

The disadvantages are:

- the model may need many time periods if the events involved are not rare.

- the 'memoryless' property. In many cases this can be overcome by disaggregation. Sonnenberg and Beck (1993) provide more information on this, and on other refinements of the basic Markov modelling approach. Disaggregation can quickly become unwieldy though. For example, in simulating prevention programmes for heart disease, the risk factors can include age, sex, blood pressure, cholesterol, smoking and more, with different combinations of these factors implying different risks. Continuous variables such as blood pressure have to be grouped to provide blood pressure categories, and a Markov model might need thousands of 'cells' (Weinstein et al. 1987). In this situation, microsimulation may be a better approach (Babad et al. 2002). You will learn about this in Chapter 11.

## Causal loops

So far you have learned about models in which the causal relationships are one-way. In many cases, as for example in your first model-building exercise in Chapter 2, it is possible to proceed by identifying a set of outcome variables, and then the immediate 'upstream' causes, and then the causes upstream of them, and so on. In that example, cost-effectiveness depended on quality of care, which depended on audit systems, etc. In the model you have just used, deaths prevented depended on the prevalence of smoking, which depended on the uptake of smoking cessation programmes.

However, in some systems there are causal links which work both ways. One familiar example is the behaviour of waiting lists for elective surgery. Figure 10.6 shows two possible graphic models of patient flows through this 'system'. In both models these flows are seen as behaving like water flowing in and out of a tank. The inflows are new referrals, the outflows are people who have had their surgery, and the numbers on the waiting list are represented by the amount of water in the tank. In the model on the left, decreasing the inflow or increasing the outflow will decrease the depth of water, i.e. the numbers waiting, and vice versa. The implication is that one way of reducing the numbers of patients waiting would be to increase the rate of surgery.

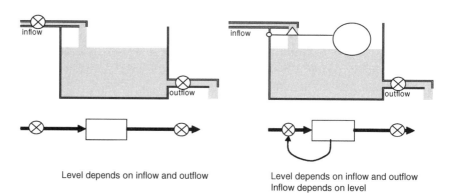

Level depends on inflow and outflow

Level depends on inflow and outflow
Inflow depends on level

**Figure 10.6** System with and without feedback

On the right of Figure 10.6 there is another model of the system. This incorporates an automatic float valve of the kind found in domestic water supplies. When the water level in the tank drops, the inflow valve opens and the flow rate increases. The result is that the level of water is kept at a reasonably constant level. By analogy, according to this model, an increase in the rate of surgery will not have a lasting effect on the numbers waiting because as the numbers waiting begin to go down, the referral rate from the community will begin to increase. The point is that although the level in the tank is affected by the inflow, the inflow is also affected by the level in the tank. This is called feedback. In this case there is a negative feedback *loop* (level down → inflow up) resulting in a *stable* system. Any 'disturbance' to the system is automatically countered and the status quo maintained.

Imagine, on the other hand, what would happen if lengthening waiting lists led to higher referral rates ('better join the waiting list now before it gets any longer'). The resulting stampede would be an example of positive feedback in action. The effect is not to counter any disturbance, but to exaggerate or amplify any small changes in the rate of inflow and destabilize the system.

Of course, in most systems there is a limit to its capacity to maintain stability. In this example, there is an upper limit on how far the inflow rates can increase, as most people are not candidates for surgery. However, these limits are often a long way away from the status quo.

This is a very simple example. Suppose you were building a macro-economic model of the health care system. It seems reasonable to suppose that utilization U will depend on morbidity M, accessibility/supply of care S and income I. However, morbidity will depend partly on utilization if health care is effective; income will depend partly on morbidity if you need to be healthy to work, and in many health care systems accessibility of care will depend on income. If so, U, M, S and I are interdependent, with relationships of the form:

$$U = a_1 + a_2 M + a_3 S + a_4 I$$
$$M = b_1 + b_2 U + b_3 I$$
$$I = c_1 + c_2 M$$
$$S = d_1 + d_2 I$$

These interdependencies imply feedback loops.

## System dynamics

One key feature of such models is the recognition that the behaviour of some parts of the system can be affected by the state of other parts, and that understanding feedback effects is important because they determine whether the response of the system as a whole to change will be stable or unstable. For example, periods of boom and bust in financial markets or population growth are widely believed to be caused by the behaviour of the various components of the system and not by exogenous factors. Most social (and biological) systems respond to disturbances – such as attempts by managers or others to change them. The premise that a system's behaviour is often a consequence of its own internal structure of feedback loops rather than external forces has led to the development of models that focus on system dynamics.

The first step in building a system dynamics model is to draw up an iconic version. This has to show how the behaviour of some parts of the system can be affected by the state of other parts. The *system boundary* separates what is considered to be inside the model (the *endogenous variables*) from what lies outside (the *exogenous variables*). The model builder will want to draw the boundary wide enough for the most important loops to be within the model. This can lead to some very broad-focus models, but the aim is generally an understanding of the system's dynamic behaviour and response to 'disturbance' rather than precise estimation.

One important feature of system dynamics iconic models is that they show both flows and effects and represent them differently. Flows appear as pipework using straight double lines and right angles, whereas effects are shown as curving single lines.

## A model with positive feedback

Consider the transmission of an infectious disease. In general, the more common the disease, the greater the risk of catching it. If a new case appears in a susceptible population, or if the incidence of the disease increases, the result is an increase in the risk of infection. This may result in a further increase in incidence and a further increase in risk of infection, and so on in a vicious circle. The feedback is positive and the resulting unstable system can create epidemics in which the disease spreads until there are not enough susceptible people left in the population to sustain it. Then it collapses.

Figure 10.7 shows a model that is also on your CD in a file called 'Ch10InfDis'. This is an infectious disease model with four states: Susceptible, Latent (infected but not yet infectious), Infectious and Resistant (immune or recovered).

This model is based on the Reed-Frost formula, $1 - (1 - p)^{I_t}$, for the risk that a susceptible individual is infected in the time slice beginning at time t, where $I_t$ is the number infected at time t. This is derived as follows: if p is the probability that two particular individuals are in effective contact during this period, then the probability that an individual avoids contact with all infectious cases in the population during this period is $(1 - p)^{I_t}$. (Effective contact means that if person A is infectious and person B is susceptible, person B becomes infected.) Also $p = R_0{}^*$length of time slice/[length of infections period*population size].

The data are in the yellow area. A few points to note:

- The model is set up to simulate a population of 100,000. Of these, 93 per cent are resistant to infection at the start of the simulation, either as a result of vaccination or having been infected at some point in the past. In this simple model, being resistant means the probability of becoming infected is zero, and resistance does not decline over time.
- The disease is not fatal but there are births and background deaths from other causes. Birth and death rates are equal, so the size of population is stable. There is no attempt to model differences between groups in the population (in terms of age or gender, say) in terms of risk of exposure or susceptibility.
- $R_0$, the basic reproduction number, is the average number of cases infected by one infectious individual in a completely susceptible population (Anderson and May 1991).

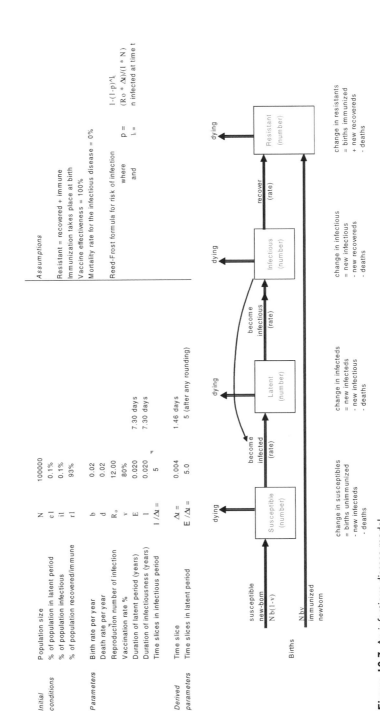

| *Initial conditions* | Population size | N | 100000 | |
|---|---|---|---|---|
| | % of population in latent period | e1 | 0.1% | |
| | % of population infectious | i1 | 0.1% | |
| | % of population recovered/immune | r1 | 93% | |
| *Parameters* | Birth rate per year | b | 0.02 | |
| | Death rate per year | d | 0.02 | |
| | Reproduction number of infection | $R_0$ | 12.00 | |
| | Vaccination rate % | v | 80% | |
| | Duration of latent period (years) | E | 0.020 | 7.30 days |
| | Duration of infectiousness (years) | I | 0.020 | 7.30 days |
| | Time slices in infectious period | $1/\Delta t =$ | 5 | |
| *Derived parameters* | Time slice | $\Delta t =$ | 0.004 | 1.46 days |
| | Time slices in latent period | $E/\Delta t =$ | 5.0 | 5 (after any rounding) |

*Assumptions*

Resistant = recovered + immune
Immunization takes place at birth
Vaccine effectiveness = 100%
Mortality rate for the infectious disease = 0%

Reed-Frost formula for risk of infection $\quad 1-(1-p)^{I_t}$
where $\quad p = (R_0 * \Delta t)/(1 * N)$
and $\quad I_t =$ n infected at time t

Susceptible (number)

Latent (number)

Infectious (number)

Resistant (number)

become infected (rate)

become infectious (rate)

recover (rate)

dying

Births

susceptible new-born
$N\,b(1-v)$

$N\,b\,v$ immunized newborn

change in susceptibles
= births unimmunized
- new infecteds
- deaths

change in infecteds
= new infecteds
- new infectious
- deaths

change in infectious
= new infectious
- new recovereds
- deaths

change in resistants
= births immunized
+ new recovereds
- deaths

**Figure 10.7** An infectious disease model

- Again, this is a Markov-type model of flow-rates between states, based on transitions over a series of time slices of equal length $\Delta t$. The user specifies the ratio (duration of infection)/$\Delta t$, which has to be a whole number, and the model calculates $\Delta t$, which is set up initially as 0.004 years (about 1.5 days).
- Once a person has become infected, they spend the next $E/\Delta t$ time slices in the 'latent' state, apart from the very small number who die from other causes. $E/\Delta t$ is calculated by the model and rounded to give a whole number. Thus, the number of people becoming infectious in any given period is the number who became infected $E/\Delta t$ periods ago, less a small number of deaths. Then they spend $I/\Delta t$ periods in the 'infectious' state. The survivors then enter the 'resistant' state, and remain there until they die.
- To get the model started, there have to be people in the latent and infectious states, and the numbers of these have to be specified by the modeller as 'initial conditions'. For this reason the formulae for the first few periods are different from the rest. In this model there is a 'run-in' period in rows 42 to 61, and these have been hidden in the spreadsheet, but if you want to see them, block-mark rows 41 to 62 in the left margin, right-click and select 'Unhide'. (The initial conditions chosen may be mutually inconsistent, in which case the model will behave erratically to start with, and will need a 'running in' period while it works its way into balance.)

 **Activity 10.5**

1 To begin with, the vaccination rate is set at 80 per cent. Try dropping this to 60 per cent, then 30 per cent, and then 0 per cent. What happens to the incidence of infection?

2 Set the vaccination rate to 40 per cent, and try reducing $R_0$. Again, what happens to incidence?

3 Set $R_0$ back to 12, and experiment with the ratio (duration of infectiousness)/(time slice $\Delta t$). Make sure that the value of $I/\Delta t$ does not exceed 10; otherwise the run-in period allowed for in constructing the model will not be long enough.

 **Feedback**

1 With a vaccination rate of 80 per cent, the incidence drops away sharply because enough of the population is resistant for the actual transmission rate of the infection to be less than 1 (i.e. on average each infected case leads to less than one new one) and the system is stable. However, with a vaccination rate of 60 per cent, there is an epidemic after six years. Enough of the population has become susceptible for the transmission rate to be above 1, and the system becomes unstable. With a vaccination rate of 30 per cent there is an epidemic after four years, and with no vaccination programme at all the interval between epidemics drops to about 2.5 years.

2 As $R_0$ drops below 8, the epidemics disappear, or at least become very infrequent. This is because if less than one-eighth of the population is susceptible, the transmission rate drops below 1 per case.

3 The frequency of epidemics appears to be reasonably robust to the choice of $I/\Delta t$, although it does increase slightly as $I/\Delta t$ approaches 1. The most noticeable change with increasing $I/\Delta t$ is that the period of time covered by a fixed number of time slices decreases, and so does the number of epidemic cycles covered.

## Summary

In this chapter you have been concerned with modelling flows around systems. You started by learning about tree models, which can be useful if the outcomes of interest occur within a narrow time band at some fixed period after intervention. If not, one approach is to divide time into a sequence of slices. In recursive tree models, each final branch in one time slice may become the trunk of a new tree in the next slice, but this approach becomes unwieldy very quickly if there are many branches and time slices. Markov models avoid this proliferation by assuming the 'memoryless' property (that the probability of changing from state A to state B in a given time slice depends only on A and B).

In some systems there are causal loops, and these determine whether the response to disturbance is stable or unstable behaviour. In system dynamics modelling the aim is to understand this behaviour or take it into account.

## References

Anderson RM and May RM (1991) *Infectious Diseases of Humans*. Oxford: Oxford University Press.

Babad H, Sanderson C, Naidoo B, White I and Wang D (2002) Modelling primary prevention strategies for coronary heart disease. *Health Care Management Science* 5: 269–74.

Doll R, Peto R, Boreham J and Sutherland I (2004) Mortality in relation to smoking: 50 years' observations on male British doctors. *British Medical Journal* 328: 1519–28.

Sonnenberg FA and Beck JR (1993) Markov models in medical decision making: a practical guide. *Medical Decision Making* 13: 322.

Weinstein MC, Coxson PG, Williams LW et al. (1987) Forecasting coronary heart disease incidence, mortality and cost: the coronary heart disease policy model. *American Journal of Public Health* 77: 1417–28.

Woolacott N, Jones L, Forbes C et al. (2002) The clinical effectiveness and cost-effectiveness of bupropion and nicotine replacement therapy for smoking cessation: a systematic review and economic evaluation. *Health Technology Assessment* 6: 16.

## Further reading

Hunink M, Glasziou P, Siegel J et al. (2001) *Decision-making in Health and Medicine: Integrating Evidence and Values*. Cambridge: Cambridge University Press.

Karnon J and Brown J (1998) Selecting a decision model for economic evaluation: a case study and review. *Health Care Management Science* 1: 133–40.

Naimark D, Krahn MD, Naglie G, Redelmeier DA and Detsky AS (1997) *Primer on Medical Decision Analysis Part 5: Working with Markov Processes. Medical Decision Making* 17: 152.

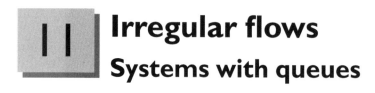

# Irregular flows
## Systems with queues

## Overview

In Chapter 11 you learned about two approaches to simulating flows in systems. Both of them involved assuming the memory-less property. Also, neither of them simulated random variation in the modelled flow rates – that is, short-term, unpredictable fluctuations that often overlay more predictable patterns of behaviour. In this chapter you will learn about another approach, microsimulation, that is not constrained in these ways and you will use it to investigate some 'what-if' questions about the number of beds in an intensive therapy unit.

This is also an opportunity to consider queues and the role of decision support systems in their management. Before going on to microsimulation techniques, you will learn how some simple queuing problems can be solved mathematically and how queuing theory can be used to make rapid estimates of mean queue length and service occupancy.

## Learning objectives

**By the end of this chapter, you will be better able to:**

- **recognize queuing systems and describe their key features**
- **define queue configuration and queue discipline**
- **give theoretical results for simple queues**
- **explain the mechanics of Monte Carlo simulation**

## Key terms

**Balking** A queuing theory term for a situation where customers are 'lost' if all servers are occupied when they arrive.

**Customers** Anyone or anything that requires a service or processing. Examples are outpatients receiving treatment, or blood samples to be tested.

**Deterministic models** Models in which it is assumed that the nature of the relationships between variables is known with certainty so that ('chaotic' systems excepted) for a given set of starting values, the results are always the same.

**Microsimulation** A method of simulation based on modelling the experience of streams of individual *entities*. Each entity can have its own set of attributes, and these may be altered during the progress of the simulation. Thus a record can be kept of an entity's 'history', and the Markov assumption is unnecessary. It is usually combined with the Monte Carlo method for sampling individuals' attributes and times to events.

**Monte Carlo method** An approach to modelling which involves using values of individual attributes and for time intervals between events that are sampled from distributions rather than fixed. Each run of the simulation gives different results and running the simulation many times gives distributions of results.

**Poisson distribution** The distribution of the number of completely random events in a given time period (e.g. the numbers of customers arriving at a service in different time periods).

**Queuing theory** Mathematical analysis that provides formulae and hence very rapid solutions for some specific queuing situations.

**Synchronous simulation** An approach to microsimulation in which time is modelled as stepping forward in periods of equal length and events occur at some indeterminate time within one of these periods.

**Stochastic models** Models in which there is an element of uncertainty about, or random variation in, at least one variable or relationship in the model. This implies an element of uncertainty about the model outputs or results, so that a series of runs provides distributions of output values.

## Flow models for queuing systems

Irregularities or fluctuations in the rates of flow of items through a system with limited capacity can have two undesirable effects:

- capacity is temporarily below the flow-rate, leading to local hold-ups or queues;
- capacity is temporarily above the flow-rate, leading to 'idle time'.

In this chapter you will learn about approaches to modelling the effects of increasing or decreasing capacity, so as to help decisions about how to strike the best balance between these two effects.

A queuing system involves the following key elements:

- *customers* – people (or objects) requiring things to be done to or for them;
- *servers or service channels* – providers of services that customers require. Typically each server or channel can serve one customer at a time.

If customers seeking a service find that there is no service channel available, they may form a queue or waiting line.

Table 11.1 gives some examples of such systems. Clearly the types of customers and services involved are all very different but, from the modelling point of view, these

**Table 11.1** Examples of queuing systems

| Example | Customers | Service channels | Typical issues |
|---------|-----------|------------------|----------------|
| intensive therapy unit | patients | beds | how many beds? |
| laboratory | specimens | machines/pathologists | batch size? |
| GP surgery | patients | general practitioners | appointments system? |
| maternity unit | mothers-to-be | beds | merge units? |
| catering | meals | nurses | delivery system? |

systems can all be represented in similar ways and can be analysed using similar methods.

The usual question in this situation is 'Where does the balance lie between providing too few service channels (an inadequate service) and too many (an inefficient one)?' Where the system is *deterministic*, with constant arrival rates and constant service times, the answer will be straightforward: if each service rate is faster than the relevant arrival rate, all will be well; and if not, queues will build up indefinitely.

However, in real systems, both arrival rates and service times will vary, usually unpredictably. In this situation, even though the average service rate is greater than the average arrival rate (so that there would be no problem in a deterministic system), there will be short periods during which the arrival rate is faster than average, and/or the service rate is slower than average. The result is that queues grow. Later, when the arrival rate drops and/or service rate increases, queues shorten again. Figure 11.1 shows how this can occur in a system with varying arrival rate but unvarying capacity.

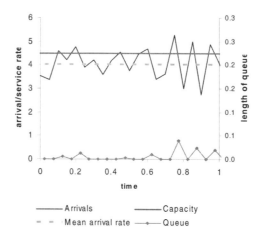

Figure 11.1 Stochastic arrivals and formation of queues

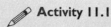 **Activity 11.1**

Queuing models provide a method of working out what capacities will be needed to provide a satisfactory service when there are irregular arrivals and/or service times. What information do you think you would need to build a model of this kind?

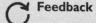 **Feedback**

To construct a queuing model you need the following information about the system:

1 *The queue configuration*: this is a description of the routes customers take between

the different services that make up the system and where the queues form. The best way of capturing this is a flow diagram.

2 *Arrival time distribution*: this is the *probability distribution* of numbers of customers arriving for a service in a given time interval. Alternatively, it can be the probability distribution of lengths of time between one customer arriving and the next. This gives an indication of how much variation there is in the arrival rate.

3 *Service time distributions*: these are the distributions of lengths of time to serve one customer at each point in the system.

4 *Queue discipline*: for each service, this covers the system of priorities that may be in operation (e.g. first come, first served); whether certain customers, or types of customers, have preferences for certain channels or types of channel; whether there is *balking*, i.e. customers who are 'lost' if a service is occupied when they arrive; and whether there is any kind of appointments system, or batching of customers.

## Queuing theory

There are two main approaches to building models of queuing problems. One involves a branch of mathematics called *queuing theory*. This provides formulae for some specific situations and hence very rapid 'solutions'. The other approach is called *Monte Carlo simulation*, which is much more flexible but can involve much more work to provide an answer.

Formulae from queuing theory are only available for a limited number of types of queuing system. In terms of queue configurations, only *simple queues* with *servers in parallel* or *servers in series* can be addressed in this way (Figure 11.2). In a simple queue with parallel servers, customers pass through only one of many similar service channels. An example might be a wound-dressing clinic in which one nurse

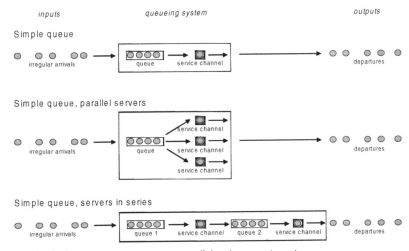

**Figure 11.2** A simple queue, servers in parallel and servers in series

is needed per patient. If there are several nurses available for this, then the clinic consists of a set of *parallel* servers. If, after having had their wounds dressed, patients have to see a receptionist to make another appointment, then the nurses and receptionists are servers in *series*.

Now define:

$$\frac{\text{mean arrival rate } (\lambda)}{\text{mean service rate } (\mu)} = \text{traffic intensity} = \rho$$

Queuing theory tells you that:

    1 the probability that a new arrival has to wait at all $= \rho$

    2 (average waiting time) / (average time in service channel) $= \rho/(1 - \rho)$

    3 average number in queue $= \rho^2/(1 - \rho)$.

These formulae depend on a number of assumptions.

1 The system is in a 'steady state', not in a period of 'transient behaviour' like the start or end of a clinic session. This means that the underlying mean arrival rates and service times are constant but subject to fluctuations about these constant values. This also implies that $\rho$ is not greater than 1. Otherwise the system will have insufficient capacity and there is no steady state as the queue will grow indefinitely.

2 The arrivals are 'random'. Each arrival is independent of other arrivals, which means that you have no knowledge other than the mean arrival rate that can help you predict when an arrival will occur. For independent identically distributed random arrivals, the variation in the number of arrivals in a given period of time can be described by a *Poisson distribution*. The shape of a Poisson distribution (named after a French mathematician) is determined by the mean arrival rate, represented by $\lambda$. Low values of $\lambda$ give distributions skewed to the right; higher values of $\lambda$ provide more symmetry. Figure 11.3 shows the shape of the distribution, and how it varies with $\lambda$.

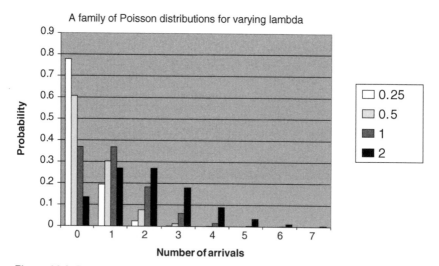

**Figure 11.3** Distribution of number of arrivals in a given period with varying lambda.

3 The variation in service times can be described by the negative exponential distribution.

One striking implication of the second of these formulae can be seen in Figure 11.4, in which (average waiting time)/(average time in the service channel) is plotted against traffic intensity. It can be seen that as traffic intensity rises above about 80 per cent, waiting times climb very rapidly in relation to time being served. This is sometimes called the 80 per cent rule. It can also be seen that if service rates are constant, the performance of the system improves, in the sense that traffic intensity can rise to nearer 90 per cent before waiting times become really long. The same is true if inter-arrival times are constant but service times follow a negative exponential distribution. As you might expect, the greater the variability in arrival and service times, the worse the performance of the system.

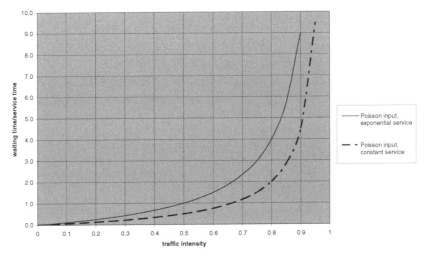

**Figure 11.4** Effect of increasing traffic intensity for different types of system

## Some rules of thumb from queuing theory

Here are some rules of thumb from queuing theory:

more randomness → longer queues for same $\rho$

priority to groups with low average service times → lower overall average queuing time.

The assumptions required by the queuing theory formulae on p. 206 (Poisson arrivals and negative exponential service times) are quite demanding, but they are of interest because they provide a 'worst-case scenario'. Other, more complex, formulae are available for other situations. For example, for a simple queue with Poisson arrivals but with service times that follow any distribution, Formula 1 above still holds, but Formula 3 becomes:

average number in queue = $[(\lambda\sigma)^2 + \rho^2]/[2*(1 - \rho)]$

where $\lambda$ is the mean arrival rate and $\sigma$ is the standard deviation of the service time.

## Parallel servers and other configurations

Formulae are also available for other more complex situations. Consider the following system with parallel service channels and balking:

- queue configuration: k parallel service channels
- arrival time distribution: Poisson, with mean arrival rate $= \lambda$
- service time distribution: any shape, but the same for all channels with mean $= \mu$
- queue discipline: balking (customers arriving when all the service channels are full cannot form a queue and are denied service).

If $\rho = \lambda/\mu$ as before, it can be shown that the probability that j out of the k channels are busy is:

$p_j = [\rho^2/j!]/\Sigma\rho^i/i!$

where $\Sigma\rho^i/i!$ is summed over the values $i = 0$ to $i = k$, and where $i! = i^*(i - 1)^*(i - 2)^* \ldots ^*1$. The most interesting case will usually be 'all channels are busy', i.e. $j = k$.

Figure 11.5 shows in graphical form some results from queuing theory on the effects of increasing numbers of parallel service channels. Results about rates of expected losses through balking are shown with solid lines in the graph and relate to the vertical scale on the left. Each line represents a different number of service channel k (3, 5, 7, 10 and 15). Corresponding results about occupancy are shown by broken lines, referred to the vertical axis on the right.

Look at the vertical line representing traffic intensity $*k = 3$. In a deterministic model, this could be managed by three channels, with 100 per cent occupancy and

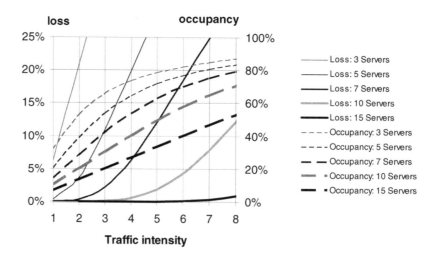

**Figure 11.5** Multi-server queues: expected losses through balking, and occupancy

no queues. Here you can see that 10 channels will give you virtually no losses through balking (solid line, k = 10, scale on left) which is good, but occupancy will be under 30 per cent (broken line, k = 10, scale on right), which is bad. Now look further up the line representing k*traffic intensity = 3. You can see that with only five channels, the probability of losses through balking increases to about 12 per cent (worse), but the occupancy increases to about 53 per cent (better). Clearly making a decision about the best number of service channels involves striking a balance between what is an acceptably high rate of losses and an acceptably low occupancy. Graphs and tables derived from queuing theory can inform such decisions.

The specialist literature provides formulae for a number of other types of queue but in general there are no formulae for circumstances where:

* customers have preferences between channels;
* there are non-random arrivals (e.g. as a result of an appointments system);
* queue configurations are complex;
* queuing systems are adaptive, e.g. when queues become long, customers are put off, and/or servers speed up (i.e. the kind of situation addressed by system dynamics models);
* the system is not in a steady state, i.e. there are changes in the underlying arrival rate and/or service time.

The simplifying assumptions needed for a queuing theory solution may be too unrealistic for the model to be a credible basis for making recommendations. Realistic models of these more complex situations require computer simulation.

## Monte Carlo simulation

In the Monte Carlo technique, random variation is 'added back' by using random numbers to choose values from *distributions* of likely values. This technique was originally developed by mathematicians interested in 'random walks', legendarily characterized as how far will a drunk be from the lamp-post after a given number of irregular zigzags. Monte Carlo *microsimulation* models set out to imitate the behaviour of the real-life system in a form of virtual reality. Rather than modelling flows as homogeneous, or deriving formulae based on summary statistics such as mean arrival and service times, the simulation model is a virtual world in which imaginary customers have imaginary attributes and histories, arriving and leaving at imaginary times, occupying and moving between imaginary service channels. There are computer software packages to help with this.

One approach to simulation is to divide time into equal short periods and move forward one period at a time, in a similar way to a Markov model. This is called *synchronous* simulation. The difference is that, while Markov processes involve splitting and merging *homogeneous groups* of people at each step, microsimulation involves modelling the progress of *individuals*.

The path through a simulation for an individual patient is shown on the left of Figure 11.6. If there are 100 people in the simulation, each will have their own pathway. Compare this with Figure 10.5 for a flow model.

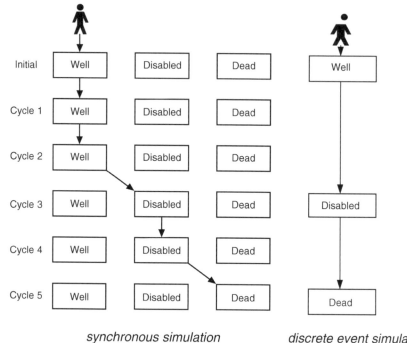

*synchronous simulation*          *discrete event simulation*

**Figure 11.6** A Monte Carlo simulation for a single patient
Source: Adapted from Sonnenberg and Beck (1993).

Now suppose that you wanted to construct a simple synchronous simulation of an Accident and Emergency Department. You would need to know:

- the distribution of numbers of new patients arriving in any given short period (15 minutes, say);
- the distribution of service times;
- the queue configuration; suppose there are two parallel treatment stations (the service channels), and when the simulation starts, station 1 is occupied for 30 minutes (the *initial conditions*);
- the queue discipline: you will assume first come, first served. To keep things simple, ignore the priority given to real emergencies.

Set the clock to a particular time, for example, 9.00 in the morning. The first step is to take a *random* sample from the distribution of numbers of new patients.

Suppose your random sample tells you that in the first 15-minute period there is one new arrival. The patient goes to the vacant treatment Station 2. Now, sampling from the distribution of service times, you find that this new patient occupies Station 2 until 10.00.

A second sample from the inter-arrival time distribution tells you that between 9.15 and 9.30 no new patients arrive. But between 9.30 and 9.45, there are two new patients. One patient can move to the now-vacant Station 1, but the other must wait until Station 2 becomes available at 10.00.

This process of sampling from arrival and service time distributions is repeated a large number of times. If the process goes on for long enough, the distributions of arrival and service times in the simulation will be very similar to those sampled from, which in turn may be based on observations in the real world. This allows you to build up a picture of what proportion of 'arrivals' have to wait for treatment, the distribution of waiting times, and how much idle time there is likely to be in the service channels. If the results match your real-world observations, you gain confidence in the model and may then use it to explore the implications of *changes* in arrival times, services times, numbers of service channels, etc.

## A paper simulation of an ITU

The best way to understand what is involved in the process described above is to try it out. In the next activity you will carry out a paper simulation of an intensive therapy unit (ITU). To make it practical without a computer, you will use rather large 'time slices' lasting one day (24 hours) each. Working through this activity will enable you to understand the elements of synchronous microsimulation and provide a basis for learning about discrete event simulation.

The configuration of the system is shown in Figure 11.7. There is no queue or waiting list for the ITU. If the ITU is full when a patient arrives, then he or she is admitted to a general hospital ward. Thus this is a queue with 'balking'.

Data for the daily number of arrivals at an ITU are shown in Table 11.2. You may assume for this exercise that the underlying mean rate of arrivals does not vary with time of day or day of the week, although of course it will do in practice. Also there is no long-term trend up or down in the underlying rate. The basic distribution is given by the column headed 'Probability'. Ignore the other columns for the time being.

Data for lengths of stay on the unit are given in Table 11.3. Again you may assume that the underlying mean stay in the unit does not vary with time of day or day of

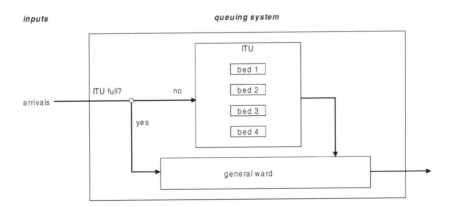

**Figure 11.7** The configuration of the ITU system

**Table 11.2** The number of arrivals per day

| Number of arrivals per day | Probability | Cumulative probability | Range of random numbers |
| --- | --- | --- | --- |
| 0 | 0.5 | 0.5 | 00–49 |
| 1 | 0.34 | 0.84 | 50–83 |
| 2 | 0.12 | 0.96 | 84–95 |
| 3 | 0.04 | 1 | 96–99 |

**Table 11.3** The length of stay (service time) in days

| Length of stay in days | Probability | Cumulative probability | Range of random numbers |
| --- | --- | --- | --- |
| 1 | 0.4 | 0.4 | 00–39 |
| 2 | 0.35 | 0.75 | 40–74 |
| 3 | 0.25 | 1 | 75–99 |

the week, and there is no long-term trend. The other columns will also be described later in the text.

You are going to simulate two weeks of admissions and departures from the ITU. To help you do this, two columns have been added to Tables 11.2 and 11.3. The probabilities in each row have been used to form cumulative probability distributions, and these in turn have been used to define ranges of random numbers. For example, in the long run, 50 per cent of the random numbers from a uniform distribution between 0 and 99 will lie between 0 and 49; 34 per cent of them will lie between 50 and 83, etc. (A uniform distribution in the range 0 to 99 means that every number between 0 and 99 has an equal chance of being selected.)

These tables allow you to convert random numbers into a number of arrivals for each day. Suppose your random number is 49. The first line in the table tells you that this corresponds no new arrivals. A number between 50 and 83 corresponds to 1 new arrival, and so on. The principle that underlies Monte Carlo simulation is that if you do this for enough random numbers and time intervals the distribution of arrival rates will match the probability distribution in Table 11.2.

## Activity 11.2

To carry out the simulation, work though the following steps:

1   Use the random number 'stream' given in Table 11.4 and the distribution in Table 11.2 to determine the number of patients arriving on the next day. In this example, the first random number is 89 and this lies in the range 84–95, which corresponds to 2 arrivals for day 1. (You could choose your own 'stream' of random numbers from a published table or generate one using the RAND() function in your spreadsheet software but this would give you slightly different answers.)

**Table 11.4** Random numbers to determine the number of arrivals per day

| Random number | 89 | 91 | 13 | 43 | 72 | 63 | 97 | 57 | 86 | 33 | 55 | 39 | 14 | 89 |
|---|---|---|---|---|---|---|---|---|---|---|---|---|---|---|
| Number of arrivals | 2 | | | | | | | | | | | | | |

2  Use the random numbers in Table 11.5 and the distribution in Table 11.3 to determine the length of stay of each new arrival. You have 2 arrivals on day 1 so you need 2 random numbers, 53 and 75, and these correspond to lengths of stay of 2 and 3 days respectively.

**Table 11.5** Random numbers to determine length of stay for each patient

| Random number | 53 | 75 | 12 | 45 | 90 | 53 | 28 | 64 | 07 | 21 | 13 | 99 | 47 | 03 | 47 | 31 |
|---|---|---|---|---|---|---|---|---|---|---|---|---|---|---|---|---|
| Length of stay | 2 | 3 | | | | | | | | | | | | | | |

3  Mark the lengths of stay in the chart (Figure 11.8) by shading in or crossing off the appropriate number of squares. Each square corresponds to one day. The 2 arrivals on the first day have been shaded in for you with lengths of stay 2 and 3 days.

| | | Week 1 | | | | | | | Week 2 | | | | | | |
|---|---|---|---|---|---|---|---|---|---|---|---|---|---|---|---|
| Day | | 1 | 2 | 3 | 4 | 5 | 6 | 7 | 1 | 2 | 3 | 4 | 5 | 6 | 7 |
| Number of arrivals | | 2 | | | | | | | | | | | | | |
| Length of stay | 1 | 2 | | | | | | | | | | | | | |
| | 2 | 3 | | | | | | | | | | | | | |
| | 3 | | | | | | | | | | | | | | |
| Bed 1 | | ▓ | ▓ | | | | | | | | | | | | |
| Bed 2 | | ▓ | ▓ | ▓ | | | | | | | | | | | |
| Bed 3 | | | | | | | | | | | | | | | |
| Bed 4 | | | | | | | | | | | | | | | |
| Number of beds occupied | | 2 | | | | | | | | | | | | | |
| Number of balked patients | | 0 | | | | | | | | | | | | | |

**Figure 11.8** Chart for recording events and performance in a discrete event simulation

4  Move forward one day, go back to step 1 of this Activity and repeat these four steps until you have completed two weeks.

Notice that this implies that the unit was empty at the beginning of the simulation. If you are unhappy about this you could put in one or two patients with 1 or 2 days stay remaining. Doing this, which is called setting up the initial conditions, can be arbitrary but the usual approach is to run the simulation for a long time so that the initial conditions have no material effect on the results.

You must allocate new admissions to the available beds in the order in which they were sampled, so that the patient whose length of stay was determined first must be added to the chart first. If one or more arrivals cannot be admitted because all the beds are full, make a record of how many in the row marked 'Number of balked patients'.

**Feedback**

The completed simulation using the random number streams given is shown in Figure 11.9.

| | Week 1 | | | | | | | Week 2 | | | | | | |
|---|---|---|---|---|---|---|---|---|---|---|---|---|---|---|
| Day | 1 | 2 | 3 | 4 | 5 | 6 | 7 | 1 | 2 | 3 | 4 | 5 | 6 | 7 |
| Number of arrivals | 2 | 2 | 0 | 0 | 1 | 1 | 3 | 1 | 2 | 0 | 1 | 0 | 0 | 2 |
| Length of stay    1 | 2 | 1 | | | 3 | 2 | 1 | 1 | 1 | | 2 | | | 1 |
|    2 | 3 | 2 | | | | | 2 | 3 | | | | | | 2 |
|    3 | | | | | | | 1 | | | | | | | |
| Bed 1 | | | | | | | | | | | | | | |
| Bed 2 | | | | | | | | | | | | | | |
| Bed 3 | | | | | | | | | | | | | | |
| Bed 4 | | | | | | | | | | | | | | |
| Number of beds occupied | 2 | 4 | 2 | 0 | 1 | 2 | 4 | 2 | 2 | 1 | 2 | 1 | 0 | 2 |
| Number of balked patients | 0 | 0 | 0 | 0 | 0 | 0 | 1 | 0 | 0 | 0 | 0 | 0 | 0 | 0 |

**Figure 11.9** Completed hand-simulation chart for a four-bedded ITU

 **Activity 11.3**

Use the completed simulation in Figure 11.9 to calculate:

1 the probability that an arriving patient is balked;
2 the proportion of beds occupied over the two-week period.

 **Feedback**

One person is balked (on day 7 of week 1) out of 15 arrivals over the two-week period so your estimate of the probability that an arrival is balked is 1/15. There are 14 × 4 = 56 bed-days available during this 14-day period. Of these, 25 were occupied (25 shaded squares). So your estimate of bed occupancy is 25 / 56 = 44.6 per cent.

 **Activity 11.4**

How reliable do you think these estimates are?

 **Feedback**

These estimates are based on a single very short simulation run. Each random number stream will be different and the result of each run will be different. In practice, many simulation trials are performed and the results averaged to obtain a more accurate result.

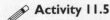

**Activity 11.5**

What do you expect would happen if there were only two beds in the ITU (admittedly rather an extreme case)?

**Feedback**

A simulation model could be used to assess the effect of reducing the number of beds in the ITU to 2. The results of this 'what-if' calculation are shown in Figure 11.10. For this configuration and this simulation run, the estimate for the probability of being balked is 5/15 = 33 per cent, and for the bed occupancy is 19/28 = 67.9 per cent.

| | | Week 1 | | | | | | | Week 2 | | | | | | |
|---|---|---|---|---|---|---|---|---|---|---|---|---|---|---|---|
| Day | | 1 | 2 | 3 | 4 | 5 | 6 | 7 | 1 | 2 | 3 | 4 | 5 | 6 | 7 |
| Number of arrivals | | 2 | 2 | 0 | 0 | 1 | 1 | 3 | 1 | 2 | 0 | 1 | 0 | 0 | 2 |
| Length of stay | 1 | 2 | 1 | | | 3 | 2 | 1 | 1 | 1 | | 2 | | | 1 |
| | 2 | 3 | 2 | | | | | 2 | | 3 | | | | | 2 |
| | 3 | | | | | | | 1 | | | | | | | |
| Bed 1 | | | | | | | | | | | | | | | |
| Bed 2 | | | | | | | | | | | | | | | |
| Number of beds occupied | | 2 | 2 | 1 | 0 | 1 | 2 | 2 | 1 | 2 | 1 | 2 | 1 | 0 | 2 |
| Number of balked patients | | 0 | 2 | 0 | 0 | 0 | 0 | 3 | 0 | 0 | 0 | 0 | 0 | 0 | 0 |

**Figure 11.10** Completed hand-simulation chart for a two-bedded ITU

In this simulation of a two-bedded unit, the same two random number streams have been used as in the earlier simulation of the four-bedded unit, one stream for arrival times and one for service times. Using different random number streams for different parameters in this way helps to ensure that differences in the results between different simulation 'runs' are mainly due to the change in configuration rather than using different sets of random numbers. Two random number streams were used because if you had used only one stream for sampling both service and arrival times, taking the next random number off the list every time you needed one, some random numbers that were used for service times in the first simulation would have been used for arrival times in the second, and vice versa. This would have made the results more difficult to compare. Again, more simulation 'runs' should be used to obtain more reliable estimates.

## Event-driven simulation

This paper simulation demonstrated the principles of Monte Carlo sampling using the *synchronous* method of dividing time into a series of slices of equal duration – a day in this case – and moving forward in time in a series of equal steps.

In computer simulation, the more usual approach is *event-driven*, mainly for reasons of computational efficiency. In the ITU simulation, arrivals and departures from the unit would be the *events*. You would sample from a continuous distribution of *inter-arrival* times, so that instead of three patients arriving within a 24-hour period, there might be *arrivals* at 09.30, 16.20 and 20.40. With lengths of stay of, say, 10.30, 35.20 and 27.50 hours there would be, in chronological order, *departures* at 20.00, 48.30 and 51.40.

In the paper-based simulation of an intensive care unit that you have just done, time was divided into slices of equal length: 24 hours. Now you will use a Excel-based discrete-event simulation model.

Open the file 'Ch11ITUSim' on your CD and familiarize yourself with the model on the worksheet called 'Simulation'. The yellow area to the top left of the worksheet contains the following data:

- the defining parameters for the inter-arrival time distribution (lengths of time between successive new arrivals);
- the defining parameters for the service time distribution;
- the queue configuration.

The two distributions are both of the gamma type. This is a family of distributions defined by two parameters: scale and shape. (Some examples are given on the sheet called 'Gamma' in Ch11ITUSim.)

### Inter-arrival times

On 'Simulation', notice that the mean inter-arrival time is 0.7 (cell D6). This is equivalent to the mean arrival rate = 10/7 you had in the paper-based simulation. The shape parameter for the inter-arrival distribution has been set to 1. This is a special case of the gamma distribution and gives a negative exponential distribution, i.e. completely random arrivals, again the same as for the paper-based simulation. You can see the shape of the distribution in the first chart on the right of the spreadsheet. Try experimenting with changing the mean (in cell D6) and shape parameter (in F6); this diagram shows you the effects on the distribution, but put back the original values before you start simulating. (Don't try and change the scale parameter because this is derived by formula from the mean and shape.)

### Service time

In this case the shape parameter is much greater than 1. This gives a distribution that is nearer Normal, although somewhat skewed to the right, again similar to the paper-based version. You can see the shape of the distribution in the second chart on the right of the spreadsheet. Again, experiment with changing the parameters, but put back the original values (1.5 and 5) before moving on to the next step. This is an example of the flexibility of the gamma distribution (also known as the Erlang distribution if the shape parameter > 1) after a Danish pioneer of queuing theory who used it in the design of telephone exchanges.

## Queue configuration

This is set up as a three-bedded unit with balking. You can change the number of beds in cell D10, but not the queue discipline.

## Initial conditions

The simulation is currently set up to have two patients in it at the start of the run, with some time remaining before they are discharged (set in cell D14). You can change this if you like.

## Model outputs

In the middle of the spreadsheet there is a pale blue area. This provides the model outputs which are defined in the same way as for the paper-based simulation:

- percentage occupancy
- percentage turned away.

It also provides the means of the inter-arrival and service times actually sampled during the simulation.

## The model

In the lower part of the screen, in the rusty orange-coloured area, is the actual simulation. This is equivalent to your worksheets in the paper-based simulation. However, instead of columns representing time slices, in this case you have a row for each new arrival time. You can see by scrolling down the page that you are simulating 1000 new arrivals (patients 3 to 1002; according to the 'initial conditions', patients 1 and 2 are in the unit when the simulation starts). Some cells have comments attached which explain the formulae involved.

### Columns C to H

This is where the inter-arrival and service times are generated, and the time of departure from the unit calculated. Use your cursor to have a look at the formulae that lie behind each cell in the first row in the body of the table, row 25. You can see that the Excel function RAND() has been used to generate random numbers and GAMMAINV(random value, alpha, beta) to sample values from the inverse of the gamma distribution (which is what you have to do to get a gamma-shaped frequency distribution).

### Columns J to O

These show, at the time each patient arrives, which beds are occupied and when the occupant of each bed is due to leave. Column J deals with bed 1. If the time of departure of the person in bed 1 is later than this arrival time, (i.e. J25 > E26), he or she is still there in row 26.

Columns K to O deal with the other beds, up to maximum of six altogether. The formulae here are more complicated. For example, column M shows activity in the 4th bed in the unit. If there are only three beds in the unit (i.e. M$22 > D$10) a blank [char(32)] is placed in the cell. If the person in it is due to leave after this new person arrives (e.g. M25 > E26), his or her leaving time is still there in row 26. If this bed is empty however, you put the leaving time of the new arrival in this bed *unless* you have already put the new arrival in another bed. You check this by using (MATCH($H26,$J26:L26,0)), i.e. does the value in H26 match any value in the set of cells J26 to L26?

## Check the model

First, have a close look at the first few rows. Does the model appear to be working as it should be?

Next, check whether the Monte Carlo sampling processes have been set up correctly. The simulated and actual gamma distributions for inter-arrival and service times are given in the worksheet called 'Evaluation'. To run a simulation press F9. Each time you do this, a different set of random numbers is used. Run it a few times and you will see how the simulated distribution is slightly different each time. But are they reasonably similar to the theoretical distribution each time?

This spreadsheet is set up to do model runs of 1000 arrivals. Is this enough? Are the differences between runs big enough to worry you about the reliability of the resulting estimates of occupancy and loss rate? One way of checking this is to look at the running plots (the two graphs on the right-hand side of the spreadsheet) on 'Evaluation'. In these the estimates of the outcomes (occupancy and balking) after n arrivals have been simulated and plotted against n. You can see that there can be quite wide swings in estimated values in the early stages of the simulation when n is small, but that as the numbers of arrivals in the simulation increase, these oscillations die down. In fact, the cumulative values change very little after about 500 arrivals.

There is another check that you can do in this case because, as it happens, the problem is of a form that can be solved exactly by queuing theory. So you can check the results for occupancy and numbers of patients lost against the formula given earlier:

$p_i = [\rho^2/j!]/\Sigma\rho^i/i!$

The calculations are given in the spreadsheet called 'Theoretical'. To make this task even easier, the results in this table for the number of beds in the current simulation are also shown in cells U4 and U29 of 'Evaluation'. Are the simulated and theoretical values similar?

(Of course, for most problems you would not be able to check your results against theory in this way because there is no theoretical solution available. And for most purposes, if there is a theoretical solution, there is not much point in solving by simulation!)

## Using the model

You want to examine the effect of changing the numbers of beds on the occupancy and balking. To do this you should complete the Results table, which you can find in Ch11ITUSim by clicking on the tag with the label 'Results – empty table'.

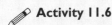 **Activity 11.6**

Set the model up with one bed and copy the figures for occupancy and loss rate into the appropriate columns of 1st row of the table headed 'run 1'. (Remember to copy using Paste Special/Values.) Run the model with one bed again by pressing the function key F9 and copy the outcomes in the Results table in the column headed 'run 2'. Repeat and copy into 'run 3'.

Now set the model up with two beds and copy the performance figures into the 2nd row of the table in the column headed 'run 1' and repeat for 'run 2' and 'run 3'.

Repeat for 3, 4, 5 and 6 beds. Now you have three values for occupancy and three for percentage balked, for each number of beds. You will see that the answers are a little different each time; how different they are tells you something about the precision of your estimates from each run.

Compare the results from the Excel simulation with those from your hand simulation. They should be broadly similar but the Excel simulation results will generally be much more accurate because you have simulated 1000 rather than about 40 arrivals.

 **Feedback**

Look at the table called 'Results – data' in Table 11.6. You will not get exactly the same results as those shown in this table because different random number streams will have been involved, but you should be reasonably close. The trade-off between occupancy and balking is clear.

**Table 11.6** Occupancy and percentage loss for different sizes of unit

| Number of beds | % occupancy | | | | | % loss | | | | |
|---|---|---|---|---|---|---|---|---|---|---|
| | run 1 | run 2 | run 3 | mean | std | run 1 | run 2 | run 3 | mean | std |
| 1 | 68.8 | 68.6 | 68.3 | 68.6 | 0.25 | 67.3 | 69 | 68.9 | 68.4 | 0.95 |
| 2 | 58.7 | 61.2 | 62.7 | 60.9 | 2.02 | 41.2 | 43.3 | 42.6 | 42.4 | 1.07 |
| 3 | 53.7 | 57.2 | 54.5 | 55.1 | 1.83 | 23.5 | 21.4 | 20.2 | 21.7 | 1.67 |
| 4 | 48.8 | 49.6 | 47.5 | 48.6 | 1.06 | 11.8 | 11.7 | 10.8 | 11.4 | 0.55 |
| 5 | 41.5 | 44.7 | 40.8 | 42.3 | 2.08 | 4.3 | 5.1 | 4.3 | 4.6 | 0.46 |
| 6 | 36.0 | 36.6 | 35.8 | 36.1 | 0.42 | 2.1 | 1.8 | 4.3 | 2.7 | 1.37 |

## Adding in system dynamics

So far it has been assumed that the average service time is constant, although subject to random fluctuation. However, it seems quite plausible that when the arrival rate is high and patients start being turned away, the processes of care might be speeded up. Extra staff might be brought in or patients might be discharged relatively early. If this is the case, a period of high occupancy will lead to temporarily low service times. When the occupancy drops and the pressure is off, the processes of care may slow down and services times increase. If so, the system includes a *negative feedback* loop which will tend to keep occupancy rates more even than they would be in a system without feedback. Another possibility is that when things get busy, the smooth running of the unit is disrupted and service times actually increase. This would be positive feedback.

Are these possibilities that you should worry about in your analysis? This is a question that simple queuing theory cannot answer but your spreadsheet can. There are four parameters that you have not used yet in the yellow 'inputs' area of 'Simulation'. Under the heading 'Feedback' in cell G9, these are 'target occupancy', 'direction', 'scale' and 'smoothing'.

It is assumed that there is a target occupancy, set initially at 50 per cent (cell H10). The system responds to periods of occupancy above this level by reducing mean service times, and to periods below this level by increasing mean service times.

'Direction' specifies whether the system is subject to negative or positive feedback and can only take the values – or +. You can change this using a drop-down menu.

'Scale' can take any value between 0 (no feedback) and 5 (maximum feedback). If you try to put in a value outside this range, you will get a message telling you that 'the value you entered is not valid'. This was set up using Excel's Data/ Validation screen. In the simulations you have run so far, this parameter has been set to zero.

'Smoothing' can take any value between 0 and 1. The lower the smoothing constant, the longer the period the system takes into account when applying feedback and the greater the smoothing effect. It may be a very short-term response, i.e. full-scale feedback is applied if occupancy is above target level for just one period. Or it may be slower to react, with some sort of moving average process to smooth out variations in occupancy rate.

The effect of feedback in this model is to multiply the scale parameter for the service time distribution by the amount in column AB. Try a run with negative feedback and compare the figures in column U on the 'Evaluation' spreadsheet for 'From simulation' with those for 'Theoretical with actual traffic intensity'. You can see that loss rates are lower than they would have been without feedback, especially with relatively large-scale feedback and strong smoothing (i.e. small smoothing constant). However, the occupancies also drop overall, because there are shorter lengths of stay in busy periods even when this would not have avoided any balking. Positive feedback, on the other hand, leads to high occupancy but far more patients being turned away. Increasing the occupancy target does increase occupancy, but to get near the target requires large-scale feedback and weak smoothing (large smoothing constant) and is linked to substantial increases in loss rate.

You can see from this how such a model might be used to explore the effects of possible adaptive responses.

## Some uses and advantages of microsimulation

Although originally developed in the context of complex queuing problems in which irregular flows are the key feature, microsimulation has been used in a much wider range of applications than this. The method can be used to model almost any type of system and it is one of the modeller's most powerful techniques, partly because it requires fewer simplifying assumptions than other methods.

In the context of irregular flows you have seen that it has a number of advantages over queuing theory:

- distributions do not have to follow specific theoretical forms but can be based on direct observation;
- appointment systems, priority schemes and complex configurations can all be accommodated;
- systems do not have to be in a steady state.

Microsimulation involves the creation of 'entities' (patients, laboratory specimens, etc.) that flow through the system and these entities can be assigned attributes, including how long they have spent in earlier states. Different distributions of service times or of times to a change in health status for example, can then be used, depending on these patient attributes.

The implication is that in the context of smooth flows:

- microsimulation methods have the advantage over Markov processes and system dynamics of not requiring the 'memory-less' or 'homogeneous flows' assumption;
- it is relatively easy to include resource constraints.

Also, the very direct way that it imitates the real world makes it a relatively transparent approach. In particular, the design of some recent software has paid a good deal of attention to having a friendly user interface, so that:

- It is relatively easy to alter model parameters, and 'what if' experiments can be set up rapidly.
- Problem-owners can see what features of the real world a model does incorporate and what features it leaves out. Some packages include animation facilities so that users can see on their computer screen how patient 'icons' move between services and how queues build as the simulation progresses. Computer games are very particular types of simulation, and sooner or later some of the techniques involved in their development will spill over into this field.

### What are the drawbacks?

In some ways it is a disadvantage that with different random number streams each simulation run will produce a slightly different result. It is possible to estimate the scale of variation of this kind, but this requires repeated runs (Davies and Davies

1994). At the same time this variability is one of the advantages of the approach, as it provides an indicator of the amount of imprecision in the results arising from actual variation in the population in sampled attributes such as blood pressure or treatment cost. (This is not the same as the variability of outputs provided by add-ins such as @RISK in a Markov model, which indicates the effect of imprecision in estimated *mean values* of parameters such as blood pressure or treatment cost.)

Because the approach is so flexible, it is tempting to put more detail into the model than is strictly necessary for the purpose in hand – although some secondary detail may be needed for credibility among problem-owners.

In the past, microsimulation has involved dedicated programming. More recently simulation software has become available at an affordable price, but in general this has been more suited to dealing with queuing problems than health care policy analysis. Dedicated programming is time-consuming, costly and prone to error, and long periods can elapse between recognition of the need for a model and a fully debugged version becoming available. Such models need to be very well documented because programmers change jobs. Also complex simulation models can take a good deal of computer time to run, and this may limit how much model testing and sensitivity analysis actually gets done, but hardware developments have been and will continue to be helpful here.

## Summary

You have learned about some of the elements of queuing theory and how this can be used to gain insight into queuing management problems such as the trade-off between bed occupancy and queue size.

You also learned that microsimulation models can be used for queuing problems where it is not possible to formulate an analytical queuing theory model, and also for a wide variety of other purposes. They do not depend on the Markov assumption, and running them many times provides an estimate of the variability of outcomes that can be expected because of the variability of key attributes in the population. However, they can be expensive to build and may require a lot of computer time.

## References

Davies R and Davies HTO (1994) Modelling patient flows and resource provision in health systems. *Omega, International Journal of Management Science* 22: 123–31.
Sonnenberg FA and Beck JR (1993) Markov models in medical decision-making: a practical guide. *Medical Decision Making* 13: 322.

# 12 Outline review

## Overview

The aim of this book has been to provide you with a way into methods from operational research and management science that can support management decision making in health care. To this end, it has provided a broad evaluative survey of the main concepts and some limited 'hands-on' experience with models, rather than expertise in specific techniques.

A great deal of ground has been covered and the purpose of this post-script chapter is to give you a brief but scannable overview. The format leaves no room for nuance, but it should help you see in very broad terms how the different methods and ideas relate to each other.

## Introduction

The review is arranged in three broad areas: decision making, models for resource allocation, and models for policy evaluation. For each of these areas there are several key ideas or concepts. Each key idea or concept is related to

- a type of problem, indicated by bullet points on the left
- more specific or related ideas and concepts in *italics*
- the aim or output of each technique, indicated by →.

## Clarifying complex decisions

### Many decision makers

- Differences in perception about ends and means

  Strategic Options Development and Analysis (Chapter 3)
  *Cognitive and strategic maps, strategic workshop*
  → Individual views explored/captured/shared
  → Agreement and commitment to a way forward

- Major one-off decision
- Options/scenarios need exploring

  Decision Conferencing (Chapter 6)
  *Facilitated group Decision Analysis (q.v.)*
  → Agreement and commitment to a decision

## Uncertainties ignored or addressed through sensitivity analysis

- Decision with one criterion      Marginal Analysis (Chapter 2)
  *Marginal benefit, marginal cost*
  $\rightarrow$     An optimal solution, or steps towards one
- Decision with many criteria      Performance Matrix (Chapter 4)
  *Explicit options, criteria and ratings*
  $\rightarrow$     A basis for a subjective decision or MCDA
- Decision with many criteria      Multiple Criteria Decision Analysis (Chapter 4)
  *Weighting, satisficing, sequential elimination*
  $\rightarrow$     A shortlist or a decision

## Uncertainty about outcomes taken into account

- No probabilities for scenarios      Game Theory (Chapter 5)
- One decision point      Utilities attached to outcomes
  *Payoff matrix, minimax etc.*
  $\rightarrow$     Avoid adverse outcomes or regrets

- No probabilities for scenarios      Robustness Analysis (Chapter 5)
- A series of decision points      Preferences/ratings attached to outcomes
  *Trumpet of uncertainty*
  $\rightarrow$     Identify options closing off fewest good outcomes

- No probabilities for scenarios      Strategic Choice (Chapter 5)
- Interconnected decision areas      Compatible and incompatible options
  *AIDA, decision graph, option tree*
  $\rightarrow$     A shortlist of compatible options

- Probabilities for scenarios      Decision Theory (Chapter 6)
- One or a series of decision      Utilities attached to outcomes
  points      *Decision tree*
  $\rightarrow$     Maximize expected utility

## Models for planning and allocating resources

- One care group      Needs Assessment (Chapter 7)
- Appropriate level      *Norms, coverage, evidence-based; incremental*
  $\rightarrow$     Amount of each resource/activity for given population?
- Several care groups      Programming (Chapter 8)
- Best mix of activity      *Constraints, feasible region; dependency, modes of care, coverage, quota*
  $\rightarrow$     Effect of altering resource levels on coverage, quality
- Uneven geographic distribution      Spatial Allocation models (Chapter 1, briefly)
  of population/providers      *Access, gravity models, deterrence function, referral models*
  $\rightarrow$     Effect of different geographic configurations
  $\rightarrow$     Good geographic access
- How hospital costs depend on      Hospital models (Chapter 9)
  resource and activity levels      *Cost triggers, flexible budgets, case mix, DRGs*
  $\rightarrow$     Cost implications of proposed changes
  $\rightarrow$     +/– knock-on effects in different departments

## Models for evaluating effects of changes in systems

| | |
|---|---|
| • Homogeneous flows in systems | Markov/State Transition Models (Chapter 10) |
| | *Transition probability, transition matrix; cycle tree, Markov* |
| | *property* |
| → | Forecast of system behaviour over time |
| • Flows in systems with causal | System Dynamics (Chapter 10) |
| loops | *Positive/negative feedback, stable/unstable systems* |
| → | Response to system 'disturbance' |
| • Irregular flow rates/service | Queuing Theory (and Microsimulation) (Chapter 11) |
| times | *Arrival/service time distributions, configuration, queue* |
| | *discipline* |
| → | Balance of queue size against occupancy |
| • Flows with individual variability | Microsimulation (Chapter 11) |
| • Markov property invalid/ | *Monte Carlo methods, synchronous vs discrete event* |
| unwieldy → | Forecast of system behaviour over time |

## References

Cropper S and Forte P eds (1997) Enhancing health services management: the role of decision support systems. Buckingham: Open University Press.

Rosenhead J and Mingers J eds (2001) Rational analysis for a problematic world revisited. London: Wiley.

Winston WL and Albright SC (1997) Practical management science. Belmont CA: Duxbury Press.

## Further reading

For a broader text in the field of health care, Cropper S and Forte P (1997) remains a useful source. There are many well produced books on applications in more general management; Winston and Albright (1997) is based on Excel and includes some useful software. For a review of problem structuring, Rosenhead and Mingers (2001) is the authoritative source.

# Glossary

**Balking** A queuing theory term for a situation where customers are 'lost' if all servers are occupied when they arrive.

**Chance node** A point at which a decision tree branches into a mutually exclusive set of states of nature. A chance node is usually represented by a circle.

**Cognitive mapping** A term from psychological research on perception which describes the general task of mapping a person's thinking. A cognitive map is not simply a 'word and arrow' diagram or an influence diagram; it is the product of a formal modelling technique with rules for its development.

**Constraints** Upper or lower limits on the level of a particular activity.

**Corporate needs assessment** A more or less formal process for adjusting the provision of health services in response to pressures for change from providers, central policy makers, professional bodies, patients and representatives of the public.

**Customers** Anyone or anything that requires a service or processing. Examples are outpatients receiving treatment, or blood samples to be tested.

**Decision Analysis** An approach to decision making which involves representing the problem in decision-tree form, branching at decision nodes and chance nodes. Probabilities are needed for each branch out of a chance node and utilities for each final branch in the tree.

**Decision area** Any area of choice within which decision makers can conceive of an alternative course of action that might be adopted, now or at some future time.

**Decision criteria** Characteristics used in judgements about preferences, or measures of performance, against which decision options are assessed. They usually relate to benefits or achievement of objectives; to cost or risks; and to feasibility.

**Decision node** The point in a decision tree where a decision must be made between competing and mutually exclusive policy or treatment options.

**Decision outcome** A combination of decision options and states of nature. Each 'terminal' branch of the decision tree represents an outcome.

**Decision tree** A type of model of a decision making problem with branches representing the possible decision options and states of nature.

**Deterministic models** Models in which it is assumed that the nature of the relationships between variables is known with certainty so that ('chaotic' systems excepted) for a given set of starting values, the results are always the same.

**Diagnosis related groups (DRG)** Classification system that assigns patients to categories on the basis of the likely cost of their episode of hospital care. Used as a basis for determining level of prospective payment by purchaser.

**Dominated option** A decision option that may be similar to another option in terms of some criteria but is inferior to it in others.

**Evidence-based needs assessment** A process through which the provision of health care can be responsive to the characteristics of the population served and evidence about the effectiveness and acceptability of the services in question.

**Expected utility** The benefit or satisfaction that an individual anticipates getting from consuming a particular good or service.

**Feasible region** All the possible combinations of values of a variable that are consistent with a given set of constraints.

**Feedback loop** The causal loop formed when flow rates out of a process or state influence the flow rates into it.

**Fixed cost** A cost of production that does not vary with the level of output.

**Flexible budget** A budget showing comparative costs for a range of levels of activity.

**Linear programming** An approach to finding feasible and, in particular, the best solutions when the constraints and objective function are linear.

**Lottery** A hypothetical gamble used in Decision Analysis to estimate the utility of an outcome.

**Marginal return** The additional benefit secured for an additional amount of expenditure. In general, marginal return diminishes with increasing expenditure.

**Markov process** An approach to modelling how systems behave over time based on the assumption that the probability of an object moving from one state to another in a given time period depends only on what the initial and final states are, and not on the object's 'history' of events or time spent in the initial state.

**Microsimulation** A method of simulation based on modelling the experience of streams of individual *entities*. Each entity can have its own set of attributes, and these may be altered during the progress of the simulation. Thus a record can be kept of an entity's 'history', and the Markov assumption is unnecessary. It is usually combined with the Monte Carlo method for sampling individuals' attributes and times to events.

**Models** Ways of representing processes, relationships and systems in simplified, communicable form. Iconic models are representations of how the system looks. Graphic models are essentially diagrams, often consisting of boxes and arrows showing different types of relationships. Symbolic models involve sets of formulae, representing the relationships between variables in quantitative terms.

**Monte Carlo method** An approach to modelling which involves using values of individual attributes and for time intervals between events that are sampled from distributions rather than fixed. Each run of the simulation gives different results and running the simulation many times gives distributions of results.

**Objective function** A mathematical function of the values of a variable which represents an objective to be either maximized (e.g. health gain) or minimized (e.g. cost).

**Operational research (OR)** The application of scientific methods to management decision making. The development and use of symbolic, and more recently, quali-tative models are arguably the distinctive features of the OR contribution.

**Payoff** In a single-criterion decision problem, the outcome or value of a given decision option for a given state of nature.

**Poisson distribution** The distribution of the number of completely random events in a given time period (e.g. the numbers of customers arriving at a service in different time periods).

**Population-based needs assessment** A process through which the provision of health care can be responsive to the characteristics of the population served.

**Population need for health** The gaps between actual and desired levels of health in a population.

**Population need for health care** The gaps between current levels of health in a population and the levels of health that they could enjoy if they had appropriate health care.

**Problem structuring** Methods of clarifying problems by developing a shared understanding of them among decision makers or stakeholders, and clarifying objectives and options. They draw on ideas about procedural as well as substantive rationality.

**Procedural rationality** An approach to decision making that stresses reasoning processes and procedures for taking decisions when capacities to process information, and to forecast and compare outcomes are limited.

**Queuing theory** Mathematical analysis that provides formulae and hence very rapid solutions for some specific queuing situations.

**Regret** For a given state of nature, the loss of payoff associated with a given decision option when compared with what would have been the payoff from the best decision option.

**Semi-variable costs** Costs that contain both a fixed and a variable element.

**Sensitivity analysis** Systematic exploration of how the outputs or results of a model change when the inputs, such as data and assumptions, are changed.

**States of nature** Possible combinations of events and circumstances that are beyond the control of the decision makers (i.e. determined by exogenous variables).

**Stochastic models** Models in which there is an element of uncertainty about, or random variation in, at least one variable or relationship in the model. This implies an element of uncertainty about the model outputs or results, so that a series of runs provides distributions of output values.

**Strategic Options Development and Analysis (SODA)** A problem-structuring approach designed for working with messy problems. The aim is to facilitate the process by which a team arrives at consensus and commitment to action. The cognitive maps of each member of a client team are merged to form an aggregated map called a 'strategic map'.

**Strategic workshops** Part of SODA, these involve two 'passes'. The aim of the first pass is to begin the process of participants 'taking on board' alternative views and in the second pass, focusing on specific issues, the 'rules' change, discussion is encouraged and commitment to action is sought.

**Substantive rationality** An approach to decision making represented by: recognizing the need for a decision; clarifying the objectives for a 'good' outcome; identifying possible courses of action; assessing these courses of action; and choosing the 'best' course of action.

**Synchronous simulation** An approach to microsimulation in which time is modelled as stepping forward in periods of equal length and events occur at some indeterminate time within one of these periods.

**Total (economic) cost** The sum of all costs of an intervention or health problem.

**Utility** Happiness or satisfaction a person gains from consuming a commodity.

**Variable cost** A cost of production that varies directly with the level of output.

**'What-if ?' analysis** A process in which the decision maker, analyst and model interact, exploring the implications of different decisions under different scenarios.

# Index